Algorithmic Approach
to Treatment

D1479292

Companion Book
Algorithmic Diagnosis of Symptoms and Signs

by R. Douglas Collins, M.D., F.A.C.P.

Algorithmic Approach to Treatment

R. Douglas Collins, M.D., F.A.C.P.
Diplomate, American Board of Internal Medicine
Diplomate, American Board of
Clinical Neurology
Consulting Neurologist
Lancaster Community Hospital
Lancaster, California

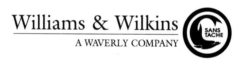

Williams & Wilkins
A WAVERLY COMPANY

BALTIMORE • PHILADELPHIA • LONDON • PARIS • BANGKOK
HONG KONG • MUNICH • SYDNEY • TOKYO • WROCLAW

351 West Camden Street
Baltimore, Maryland 21201-2436 USA

Rose Tree Corporate Center
1400 North Providence Road
Building II, Suite 5025
Media, Pennsylvania 19603-2043 USA

Library of Congress Cataloging-in-Publication Data

Collins, R. Douglas.
    Algorithmic approach to treatment / R. Douglas Collins.
        p.   cm.
    Companion v. to: Algorithmic diagnosis of symptoms
and signs / R. Douglas Collins. c1995.
    Includes index.
    1. Medical protocols—Handbooks, manuals, etc.
I. Collins, R. Douglas   Algorithmic diagnosis of
symptoms and signs.   II. Title.
    [DNLM: 1. Therapeutics. 2. Algorithms. 3. Decision
Support Techniques. 4. Cost Savings.   WB 300 C712a
1997]
RC64.C65   1997
615.5—dc21
DNLM/DLC
for Library of Congress   96-49629
                                                        CIP

ISBN: 0-683-30303-1

Printed and bound in the U.S.A.
10 9 8 7 6 5 4 3 2

Dedication

This book is dedicated to my children, Vickie, Jennifer, Paul, Douglas, Michael, Joy, and Mary Lois who have accepted JESUS CHRIST as their personal Savior.

Acknowledgments

Special recognition goes to *Clayton Reynolds, M.D., F.A.C.P., Contributing Editor, Endocrinology and Internal Medicine.*

Others who have critically reviewed the manuscript and provided many useful comments are: Enobong A. Ekong, M.D., F.A.C.C., Weiche Tsai, M.D., and Stephen Cullinan, M.D.

My wife, Norie Collins, has given me both spiritual and emotional support throughout the stages of preparation.

Finally, Melissa Pelzer is gratefully acknowledged for typing the manuscript and assistance in laying out the algorithms.

Preface

Treatment is rarely specific! The reader will quickly recall some of the diseases such as pernicious anemia, strep throat, and diplococcus pneumonia, for which we have specific therapy. By in large, however, treatment requires the deployment of *multiple therapeutic modalities* to bring about a cure. For example, a herniated disk may be managed medically with physiotherapy, anti-inflammatory drugs, and bed rest! It may also be handled surgically with a laminectomy. Often we will try one of these modalities at a time rather than costly, shotgun therapy! It behooves the clinician to not only know the various therapeutic modalities but to know which are most suitable for a specific patient at a specific period in time. He also needs to know the most cost-effective approach. For example, a patient with an acute herniated disk may require a course of conservative treatment before launching on a laminectomy that may cost several thousand dollars. A patient with coronary insufficiency may need a trial of coronary vasodilators before expensive coronary bypass surgery or angioplasty is entertained.

Algorithms lend themselves beautifully to addressing these issues! With them we can divide the patients according to their severity, the temporal relationship of the disease, their particular age, and other factors that influence our judgment.

This book is a companion to *Algorithmic Diagnosis of Symptoms and Signs*. The first book deals with diagnosis by an algorithmic approach, while this book attacks treatment by an algorithmic approach. The clinician can pick it up and at a glance get a picture of the various forms of therapy available in treating a particular disease. The clinician is also assisted in identifying when referral to a specialist is necessary or helpful. After all, referral is a form of treatment and a lot cheaper than some of the diagnostic tests we order today. Preventive therapy will be addressed where appropriate. Prognosis will be discussed in the most ominous disorders.

The author hopes that this book will fill the need for a quick handy reference for treatment, both in the office and on the hospital ward.

R. Douglas Collins, M.D., F.A.C.P.

Contents

Preface	vii
How to use this book	1
Acne	2
Acoustic neuroma	4
Actinomycosis	5
Acute abdomen, common causes	6
Adrenal insufficiency	8
Adrenogenital syndrome	9
Agammaglobulinemia, congenital	10
Agnogenic myeloid metaplasia	11
AIDS	12
Alcaptonuria and ochronosis	13
Alcoholism	14
Aldosteronism, primary	15
Allergic rhinitis	16
Alpha-1-antitrypsin deficiency	17
Alzheimer's disease	18
Amebiasis	19
Amyloidosis	20
Anthrax	21
Aortic aneurysm	22
Aplastic anemia	24
Ascaris lumbricoides	25
Asthma	26
Balantidiasis	28
Basilar artery insufficiency or thrombosis	29
Bell's palsy	30
Beriberi	31
Biliary cirrhosis	32
Blastomycosis	33
Bornholm's disease	34
Botulism	35
Brachial plexus neuropathy	36
Brain tumors, selected	37
Bronchial adenoma	39
Bronchiectasis	40
Bronchitis, acute	41
Brucellosis	42
Bursitis	43
Cancer of the stomach	44
Carbon monoxide poisoning	46

Carbon tetrachloride poisoning 47
Carbuncles and furuncles 48
Carcinoid syndrome 49
Carcinoma of the ampulla of Vater 50
Carcinoma of the breast 51
Carcinoma of the cervix 53
Carcinoma of the colon 54
Carcinoma of the endometrium 55
Carcinoma of the lung 56
Carcinoma of the ovary 57
Carcinoma of the pancreas 58
Cardiac arrest 59
Cardiac arrhythmias 61
Cardiomyopathy 63
Carpal tunnel syndrome 65
Cat-scratch disease 66
Cellulitis 67
Cerebral abscess 68
Cerebral aneurysm 69
Cerebral embolism 71
Cerebral thrombosis and infarction 73
Cervical spondylosis 74
Cervicitis 76
Chancroid 77
Cholangiocarcinoma 78
Cholangitis 79
Cholecystitis and cholelithiasis 80
Choledocholithiasis 81
Cholera 82
Choriocarcinoma 83
Cirrhosis, alcoholic 84
Coccidiomycosis 85
Conjunctivitis 87
Congenital heart disease 89
Constipation 91
Coronary insufficiency 92
Creutzfeldt–Jakob disease 95
Cryptococcosis 96
Cushing's syndrome 97
Cutaneous larva migrans 99
Cystic fibrosis 100
Cysticercosis 101
Cystinosis 102
Cystinuria 103
Cytomegalovirus infection 104
Dengue fever 105

Depression 106
Dermatomyositis 108
Diabetes insipidus 109
Diabetes mellitus 110
Diabetic coma 113
Digitalis intoxication 115
Diphtheria 116
Diphyllobothrium latum 117
Diverticular disease 118
Down's syndrome 120
Dracunculiasis 121
Dressler's syndrome 122
Drug intoxication 123
Drug reactions 124
Dubin–Johnson syndrome 125
Eaton–Lambert syndrome 126
Echinococcosis 127
Ectopic pregnancy 128
Eczema 129
Ehlers–Danlos syndrome 131
Emphysema 132
Empyema of the lung 134
Encephalitis, viral 135
Encephalomyelitis, acute disseminated 136
Eosinophilic pneumonia 137
Epididymitis 138
Epidural abscess 139
Epilepsy, idiopathic 140
Epilepsy, status 143
Erysipelas 144
Erythema multiforme 145
Erythema nodosum 146
Esophageal carcinoma 147
Esophageal varices 148
Essential hypertension 150
Extradural hematoma 152
Fabry's disease 153
Familial Mediterranean fever 154
Familial Periodic Paralysis 155
Fanconi syndrome 156
Fibromyalgia 157
Filariasis 158
Fractures 159
Fungal infections of the skin 160
Galactosemia 162
Gas gangrene 163

Gastritis	**164**
Gastroenteritis	**165**
Gaucher's disease	**167**
Giardiasis	**168**
Gilbert's disease	**169**
Gingivitis	**170**
Glanders	**171**
Glanzmann's disease	**172**
Glaucoma	**173**
Glomerulonephritis	**174**
Glycogen storage disease	**175**
Goiter, diffuse	**176**
Gonorrhea	**178**
Goodpasture's disease	**180**
Gout	**181**
Granuloma inguinale	**182**
Guillain–Barré syndrome	**183**
Hartnup disease	**184**
Head injury	**185**
Heart failure	**187**
Heat-related disorders	**189**
Hemangioblastoma	**190**
Hemifacial spasm	**191**
Hemochromatosis	**192**
Hemoglobin C disease	**193**
Hemolytic anemia, acquired	**194**
Hemophilia	**195**
Hemorrhagic fever	**196**
Hemorrhoids	**197**
Hepatitis, toxic	**198**
Hepatitis, viral	**199**
Hepatolenticular degeneration	**200**
Hepatoma	**201**
Hereditary ataxia	**202**
Hereditary elliptocytosis	**203**
Hereditary spherocytosis	**204**
Herniated disk, cervical	**205**
Herniated disk, lumbar	**207**
Herpangina	**209**
Herpes simplex	**210**
Herpes zoster	**211**
Hidradenitis suppurativa	**212**
Hirschsprung's disease	**213**
Histamine cephalalgia	**214**
Histiocytosis X	**215**
Histoplasmosis	**216**

Hookworm disease	217
Huntington's chorea	218
Hurler's syndrome	219
Hydrocephalus	220
Hypernephroma	221
Hyperparathyroidism	222
Hypersensitivity Pneumonitis	223
Hypersensitivity vasculitis	224
Hyperthyroidism	225
Hypoparathyroidism	228
Hypopituitarism	230
Hypothyroidism	232
Idiopathic postural hypotension	234
Idiopathic pulmonary fibrosis	235
Impetigo	236
Impingement syndrome	237
Infectious mononucleosis	238
Influenza	239
Insulinoma	240
Intracranial hemorrhage	241
Irritable bowel syndrome	242
Kala-azar	243
Klinefelter's syndrome	244
Korsakoff's syndrome	245
Lactase deficiency	246
Langerhans' cell granulomatosis	247
Laryngitis, acute	248
Lead intoxication	249
Legionnaires' disease	250
Leishmaniasis, cutaneous	251
Leprosy	252
Leptospirosis	253
Leriche syndrome	254
Leukemia	255
Lichen planus	257
Lipoproteinemias	258
Listeriosis	260
Liver abscess	261
Liver failure	262
Lung abscess	263
Lupus erythematosus	264
Lyme disease	265
Lymphangitis	266
Lymphogranuloma venereum	267
Lymphoma	268
Lysosomal storage disease	269

Macroglobulinemia	270
Malabsorption syndrome	271
Malaria	273
Mallory–Weiss tear	275
Marfan's syndrome	276
Mastoiditis	277
McArdle's syndrome	278
McCune–Albright syndrome	279
Meckel's diverticulum	280
Mediastinitis	281
Melanoma	282
Meniere's disease	283
Meningitis	284
Meningococcemia	286
Menopause	287
Mesenteric artery insufficiency, embolism, or thrombosis	289
Methemoglobinemia and sulfhemoglobinemia	290
Migraine	291
Milroy's disease	293
Mitral valvular disease	294
Mucormycosis	296
Multiple myeloma	297
Multiple sclerosis	298
Mumps	299
Muscular dystrophy	300
Myasthenia gravis	301
Myocardial infarction	303
Myotonia atrophica	305
Narcolepsy	306
Nephrolithiasis	307
Nephrotic syndrome, idiopathic	309
Neuroblastoma	311
Neurofibromatosis	312
Neuroma, traumatic	313
Niemann–Pick disease	314
Nocardiosis	315
Nutritional anemia	316
Obesity	318
Optic neuritis	319
Orchitis	320
Oroya Fever	321
Osteoarthritis	322
Osteogenesis imperfecta	324
Osteogenic sarcoma	325
Osteomalacia	326

Osteomyelitis 327
Osteopetrosis 328
Osteoporosis 329
Otitis externa 331
Otitis media 332
Ovarian cancer 333
Paget's disease 334
Pancreatitis 335
Panniculitis, acute 337
Paralysis agitans 338
Pellagra 340
Pemphigus vulgaris 341
Peptic ulcer 342
Periarteritis nodosa 344
Pericarditis 345
Perinephric abscess 346
Peripheral neuropathy 347
Peritonitis 350
Pernicious anemia 351
Peroneal muscular atrophy 352
Peroneal neuropathy 353
Pertussis 354
Peutz–Jeghers syndrome 355
Peyronie's disease 356
Pharyngitis and tonsillitis 357
Pharyngoconjunctival fever 358
Phenylpyruvic oligophrenia 359
Pheochromocytoma 360
Phlebotomus fever 361
Pinealoma 362
Pinworm disease 363
Pituitary adenoma 364
Pityriasis rosea 366
Plague 367
Pneumoconiosis 368
Pneumocystis carinii 369
Pneumonia 370
Pneumothorax 372
Poliomyelitis 374
Polycystic kidney disease 375
Polycystic ovary syndrome 376
Polycythemia vera 377
Polymyalgia rheumatica 378
Porphyria 379
Preeclampsia–eclampsia 380
Premenstrual tension syndrome 381

Prostatic carcinoma   382
Prostatic hypertrophy   384
Prostatitis   386
Pseudogout   387
Pseudohypoparathyroidism   388
Pseudo-pseudohypoparathyroidism   389
Pseudotumor cerebri   390
Psittacosis   391
Psoriasis   392
Pulmonary alveolar proteinosis   393
Pulmonary embolism   394
Pyelonephritis   396
Pyloric stenosis, congenital   397
Pyridoxine deficiency   398
Q-fever   399
Rabies   400
Rat-bite fever   401
Raynaud's disease   402
Reflex sympathetic dystrophy   403
Reflux esophagitis   404
Refsum's disease   405
Regional enteritis   406
Reiter's syndrome   407
Relapsing fever   408
Relapsing polychondritis   409
Renal failure, acute   410
Renal failure, chronic   412
Renal vein thrombosis   414
Retinal artery occlusion   415
Rheumatic fever   416
Rheumatoid arthritis   417
Rheumatoid spondylitis   419
Riboflavin deficiency   420
Rickets   421
Rickettsialpox   422
Rocky Mountain spotted fever   423
Rubella   424
Rubeola   425
Salmonellosis   426
Salpingitis   428
Sarcoidosis   429
Scabies   430
Scarlet fever   431
Schilder's disease   432
Schistosomiasis   433
Schizophrenia   434
Scleroderma   435

Scrub typhus   436
Scurvy   437
Seborrheic dermatitis   438
Septic arthritis   439
Septicemia   440
Serum sickness   441
Shigellosis   442
Shy–Drager syndrome   443
Sickle cell anemia   444
Sinusitis   445
Sjögren's syndrome   446
Skin cancer   447
Sleep apnea   448
Small intestinal tumors   450
Snake bite   451
Spasmodic torticollis   452
Spinal cord tumor   453
Sporotrichosis   454
Sprains, common   455
Stasis dermatitis   457
Strongyloidiasis   458
Sturge–Weber syndrome   459
Subacute bacterial endocarditis   460
Subdiaphragmatic abscess   461
Subdural hematoma   462
Syphilis   463
Syringomyelia   465
Systemic mastocytosis   466
Takayasu's disease   467
Tapeworm disease   468
Temporal arteritis   469
Testicular tumors   470
Tetanus   471
Thalassemia   472
Thoracic outlet syndrome   473
Thromboangiitis obliterans   474
Thrombocytopenia purpura, idiopathic   475
Thrombophlebitis   476
Thrombotic thrombocytopenia purpura   477
Thymoma   478
Thyroiditis, subacute   479
Tourette's syndrome   480
Toxoplasmosis   481
Trachoma   482
Transfusion reaction   483
Transient ischemic attacks   484
Trichinosis   485

Trigeminal neuralgia   **486**
Trypanosomiasis   **487**
Tuberculosis   **488**
Tuberous sclerosis   **489**
Tularemia   **490**
Turner's syndrome   **491**
Typhoid fever   **492**
Typhus, epidemic   **493**
Ulcerative colitis   **494**
Urinary tract infection   **496**
Urticaria   **498**
Uterine fibroids   **499**
Vaginitis   **500**
Varicella   **501**
Varicose veins   **502**
Variola   **503**
Venereal disease   **504**
Viral myelitis   **505**
Visceral and ocular larva migrans   **506**
Von Willebrand's disease   **507**
Warts   **508**
Wegener's granulomatosis   **509**
Wernicke's encephalopathy   **510**
Whipple's disease   **511**
Yaws   **512**
Yellow fever   **513**
Zollinger–Ellison syndrome   **514**

Index   **515**

Algorithmic Approach to Treatment

HOW TO USE THIS BOOK

There are no chapters in this book! Rather, diseases are listed in alphabetical order for easy and quick reference. The many common diseases are included, as well as most of the rare disorders.

Under each disease, the first thing to be addressed is what diagnostic test or tests should be done to confirm the diagnosis. Next, specific forms of treatment are discussed. Following that, useful alternatives are mentioned. Next, the methods of prophylaxis are indicated when possible. Finally, where it is significant, the prognosis is given. Throughout this sequence, the spots for a referral to a specialist are noted.

The algorithms and text are set up to follow the same sequence as much as possible. If there is something that is not so clear in the algorithm, it will usually be clarified in the text. Broader terms are used in the algorithms for simplicity.

The reader should be aware that these algorithms are guidelines for therapy. The actual treatment applied will vary when dealing with each individual patient. Also, each algorithm is just one way of approaching the treatment of a given disorder. Therefore, they should not be used in cookbook fashion.

Furthermore, the drug of choice, drug dosage, and other factors to be considered in treatment may change by the time the clinician gets this book in his hand. The author and publisher cannot take responsibility for these changes. Clinicians unfamiliar with the dosages and side effects of each drug must consult the current *Physician's Desk Reference*, package inserts, or standard pharmacology texts before prescribing them.

ACNE

1. Confirm diagnosis by clinical picture. Biopsy is rarely necessary.
2. *Mild to moderate cases:*
   a. Treat initially with retinoic acid (0.05 % – 0.1% Retin-A) or benzoyl peroxide cream (Fostex, etc.) and soap. Tetracycline 500 mg two to four times daily is administered orally. Alternatively, erythromycin can be given. Do not give tetracycline in pregnant women or children under 8 years old.
   b. If the above is ineffective, oral vitamin A 100,000–300,000 units may be given, and in females oral contraceptives with high-dose estrogen should be tried. Look out for vitamin A toxicity in adults.
   c. If the above is ineffective, Isotretinoin (Accutane®) should be tried. Remember, this agent is teratogenic. It is best to consult a dermatologist at this time.
3. *Severe cases:* Initial treatment is Isotretinoin (Accutane®), but consult a dermatologist for guidance.

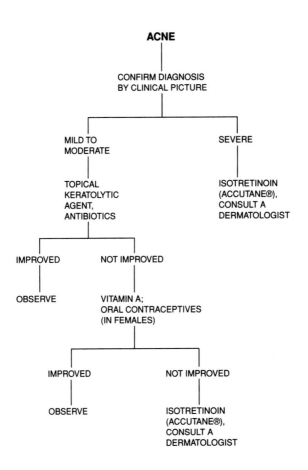

ACNE

CONFIRM DIAGNOSIS
BY CLINICAL PICTURE

MILD TO
MODERATE

SEVERE

TOPICAL
KERATOLYTIC
AGENT,
ANTIBIOTICS

ISOTRETINOIN
(ACCUTANE®),
CONSULT A
DERMATOLOGIST

IMPROVED

NOT IMPROVED

OBSERVE

VITAMIN A;
ORAL CONTRACEPTIVES
(IN FEMALES)

IMPROVED

NOT IMPROVED

OBSERVE

ISOTRETINOIN
(ACCUTANE®),
CONSULT A
DERMATOLOGIST

ACOUSTIC NEUROMA

1. Confirm diagnosis with CT scan or gadolinium-enhanced MRI. Consult a neurosurgeon.
2. *Small tumors:*
   a. If patient is over 65 years old, consider observation.
   b. If patient is under 65 years old, surgery via the transmastoid labyrinthine approach may be possible. Object is to preserve the facial nerve.
3. *Large tumors* (> 3 cm): Treat with suboccipital craniotomy or combined suboccipital and translabyrinthine approach.

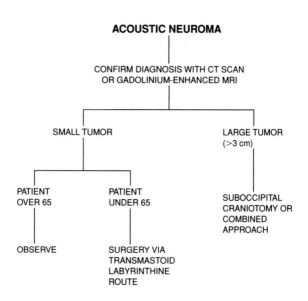

ACTINOMYCOSIS

1. Confirm diagnosis with smear and anaerobic cultures of material from infected tissue.
2. Treat with 12−20 million units of aqueous penicillin G per day for 2−6 weeks. Then switch to oral penicillin-VK 1000 mg q.i.d. for 12−18 months.
3. Alternatively, tetracycline, erythromycin, or clindamycin may be used.
4. Surgical drainage and débridement may be required in some cases.

ACUTE ABDOMEN, COMMON CAUSES

1. Confirm diagnosis with CBC, chemistry panel, serum amylase and lipase, and flat plate and upright of the abdomen.
2. Hospitalize all patients.
3. *Acute appendicitis and ruptured peptic ulcer:* Immediate surgery.
4. *Intestinal obstruction:* Treat with bowel rest, IV fluids, NG tube, and antibiotics.
   a. Patient improves. Surgery for the cause may be done after patient is stable.
   b. No improvement: Immediate surgery.
5. *Acute cholecystitis (confirm diagnosis with ultrasonography or HIDA study):*
   a. IV fluids, NG tube, antibiotics.
   b. If improvement: Surgery may be postponed until patient is stable.
   c. If no improvement: Patient should have immediate surgery.
6. *Acute pancreatitis:* Bowel rest, IV fluids, antibiotics, observation.
7. These are some of the common causes of the acute abdomen. Other causes must be kept in mind and treated accordingly.

ACUTE ABDOMEN, COMMON CAUSES

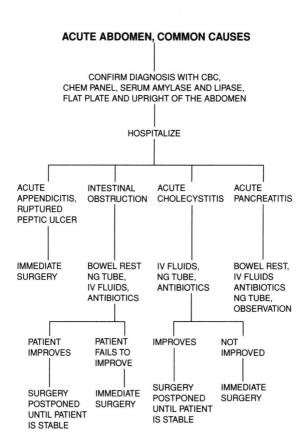

CONFIRM DIAGNOSIS WITH CBC,
CHEM PANEL, SERUM AMYLASE AND LIPASE,
FLAT PLATE AND UPRIGHT OF THE ABDOMEN

HOSPITALIZE

ACUTE APPENDICITIS, RUPTURED PEPTIC ULCER
INTESTINAL OBSTRUCTION
ACUTE CHOLECYSTITIS
ACUTE PANCREATITIS

IMMEDIATE SURGERY

BOWEL REST NG TUBE, IV FLUIDS, ANTIBIOTICS

IV FLUIDS, NG TUBE, ANTIBIOTICS

BOWEL REST, IV FLUIDS ANTIBIOTICS NG TUBE, OBSERVATION

PATIENT IMPROVES

PATIENT FAILS TO IMPROVE

IMPROVES

NOT IMPROVED

SURGERY POSTPONED UNTIL PATIENT IS STABLE

IMMEDIATE SURGERY

SURGERY POSTPONED UNTIL PATIENT IS STABLE

IMMEDIATE SURGERY

ADRENAL INSUFFICIENCY

1. Confirm diagnosis by serum cortisol, rapid ACTH test, serum ACTH level, and prolonged ACTH stimulation test. Consult an endocrinologist.
2. *Acute adrenal insufficiency:* Treat with hydrocortisone 100 mg IV q.6h. and IV dextrose and normal saline, up to 1 liter/hour until patient is stable. Monitor blood pressure and urine output and electrolytes. Use vasopressor agents, if necessary. Once patient's condition is stable, hydrocortisone dosage may be reduced gradually over 3−5 days and transferred to oral hydrocortisone. When necessary, fludrohydrocortisone 0.05−0.2 mg is given, also.
3. *Chronic adrenal insufficiency:* Treat with hydrocortisone 20−40 mg/day. Most patients also require fludrohydrocortisone 0.05−0.2 mg p.o. daily.
4. *Secondary adrenal insufficiency:* Patients usually respond to prednisone 5−30 mg q.d. Mineralocorticoids are not usually necessary. Look for and treat other secondary deficiencies (i.e., thyroid, ovarian, or testicular, etc.).

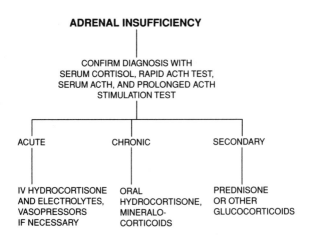

ADRENAL INSUFFICIENCY

CONFIRM DIAGNOSIS WITH
SERUM CORTISOL, RAPID ACTH TEST,
SERUM ACTH, AND PROLONGED ACTH
STIMULATION TEST

ACUTE — CHRONIC — SECONDARY

IV HYDROCORTISONE AND ELECTROLYTES, VASOPRESSORS IF NECESSARY

ORAL HYDROCORTISONE, MINERALO-CORTICOIDS

PREDNISONE OR OTHER GLUCOCORTICOIDS

ADRENOGENITAL SYNDROME

1. Confirm diagnosis with serum and urine cortisol, urine 17-hydroxy and 17-ketosteroids 17-
   hydroxyprogesterone, urine DHEA, and CT
   scans of abdomen and pelvis.
2. *Congenital adrenal hyperplasia:* Treat with
   10–30 mg of hydrocortisone and a mineralocor-
   ticoid daily. Surgical correction of the external
   genitalia may be needed. Consult an endocrinologist.
3. *Arrhenoblastoma;* Treat with oophorectomy.
   Consult a gynecologist.
4. *Adrenal carcinoma:* Treat with adrenalectomy
   and replacement therapy when possible. Treat
   with chemotherapy when resection is not possible. Consult an oncologist.

AGAMMAGLOBULINEMIA, CONGENITAL

1. Confirm diagnosis by protein and immunoelec-trophoresis and B-lymphocyte and T-lymphocyte counts.
2. Treat with intravenous immune serum globulin 400 mg/kg every 3–4 weeks.
3. Treat all infections with prophylactic antibiotics until the cause can definitely be determined not to be bacterial.
4. Consult an infectious disease specialist.

AGNOGENIC MYELOID METAPLASIA

1. Confirm diagnosis by CBC, blood smear, bone marrow biopsy, x-rays of bone, leukocyte alkaline phosphatase, and decreased red cell survival.
2. No specific therapy is available.
3. Consider bone marrow transplant. Consult hematologist.
4. Transfusions are used for anemia and pancytopenia. Consider splenectomy.
5. Chemotherapy may be useful. Consult an oncologist.

AIDS

1. Confirm diagnosis by history and demonstration of anti-HIV antibodies.
2. No specific therapy available to eradicate the virus.
3. Zidovudine (AZT) or other antiviral drug if T4 lymphocyte count falls below 500.
4. Treat opportunistic infections and malignancies. Consult infectious disease specialist.
5. Trimethoprim 160 mg and sulfamethoxazole 800 mg once daily as prophylaxis against *Pneumocystis carnii* if T4 count falls below 200.

Prophylaxis

1. No sex before marriage or out of wedlock.
2. No anal sex.
3. Use condoms and spermicidal agents.
4. Don't share needles.
5. Sex with multiple partners is forbidden.
6. Proper public health procedures of identifying and follow-up of all contacts.
7. Hepatitis B vaccine.
8. Pneumococcal vaccine.

ALCAPTONURIA AND OCHRONOSIS

1. Confirm diagnosis by urinalysis and ferric chloride test for homogentisic acid. Urine turns dark on addition of alkali.
2. No specific treatment.
3. Treat symptomatically as osteoarthritis (see page 322).

ALCOHOLISM

1. Confirm diagnosis by history, physical, blood alcohol level, and liver function tests.
2. *Acute:* Admit to alcohol unit and treat with IV fluids, long-acting benzodiazepines such as chlordiazepoxide (Librium) 25–50 mg q.4h., anticonvulsants, such as phenytoin 100 mg q.6h after loading dose, vitamins, and minerals. Haloperidol may be needed to control hallucinations. After acute stage, begin rehabilitation with group and individual psychotherapy and referral to Alcoholics Anonymous.
3. *Chronic:* Admit to alcohol unit or hospital for detoxication and follow up with rehabilitation, including group and individual psychotherapy, Alcoholics Anonymous, and so on.

ALDOSTERONISM, PRIMARY

1. Confirm diagnosis with serial electrolytes, plasma renin levels, inability to suppress aldosterone secretion, and CT scans.
2. *Adenoma:* Treat with surgical resection. Patients who are a poor surgical risk may be treated medically (see below).
3. *Hyperplasia:* Treat medically with 25–100 mg of spironolactone q.8h. If results are poor, consider subtotal bilateral adrenalectomy.
4. *Carcinoma:* These tumors should have surgery, if possible.

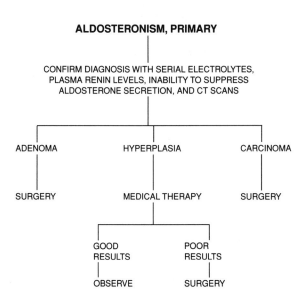

ALLERGIC RHINITIS

1. Confirm diagnosis with nasal smear for eosinophils, serum IgE level, RAST, and skin testing. Consult an allergist in difficult cases.
2. Treat initially by (a) avoiding the allergen, (b) using air filtration devices, and (c) administering H1 antihistamines such as terfenadine (60 mg b.i.d.) or astemizole. An oral decongestant may be added. Do not use intranasally.
3. If the above measures are ineffective, cromolyn sodium as a liquid nasal metered dose spray may be tried.
4. If the above is ineffective, try intranasal corticosteroids such as beclomethasone or flunisolide.
5. If all the above have been ineffective, refer to an allergist for desensitization.

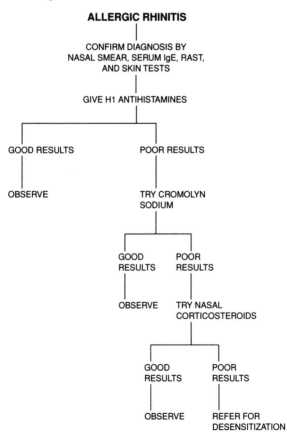

ALLERGIC RHINITIS
|
CONFIRM DIAGNOSIS BY
NASAL SMEAR, SERUM IgE, RAST,
AND SKIN TESTS
|
GIVE H1 ANTIHISTAMINES

GOOD RESULTS — POOR RESULTS

OBSERVE — TRY CROMOLYN SODIUM

GOOD RESULTS — POOR RESULTS

OBSERVE — TRY NASAL CORTICOSTEROIDS

GOOD RESULTS — POOR RESULTS

OBSERVE — REFER FOR DESENSITIZATION

ALPHA-1-ANTITRYPSIN DEFICIENCY

1. Confirm diagnosis by low levels of serum alpha-1-antitrypsin.
2. Treat with 60 mg/kg of alpha-1-antitrypsin weekly.
3. Treat the associated emphysema symptomatically (see page 132).

ALZHEIMER'S DISEASE

1. Confirm diagnosis by CT scans and MRIs.
2. Treatment is symptomatic since no specific therapy is available.
3. Recent introduction of the acetylcholinesterase inhibitor tetrahydroaminoacridine (Cognex) has allowed improvement in mental status, but liver toxicity has limited its usefulness.

AMEBIASIS

1. Confirm the diagnosis by stools for ovum and parasites, sigmoidoscopy and biopsy, and serologic tests.
2. *Intestinal amebiasis:*
   a. Asymptomatic: If the patient is seropositive, treatment with a luminal agent such as iodoquinol (650 mg t.i.d. × 20 days) or paromomycin (500 mg t.i.d. × 10 days) is advisable.
   b. Symptomatic: Begin treatment with metronidazole 750 mg t.i.d. for 5–10 days and follow with a luminal agent (see above).
3. *Amebic abscess of the liver:*
   a. Treat with metronidazole as above.
   b. If good response, follow with a luminal agent (see above for dosage).
   c. If poor response, consider aspiration or surgery. Consult an infectious disease expert and a surgeon.

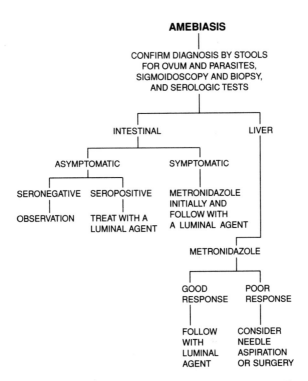

AMYLOIDOSIS

1. Confirm diagnosis by tissue biopsy (abdominal subcutaneous fat pad aspirate, rectum, liver, etc.).
2. No specific therapy is available.
3. The combination of prednisone and melphalan (or prednisone, melphalan, and colchicine) may prolong life. Consult an expert in this disease for guidance in therapy.

ANTHRAX

1. Diagnosis by history, smear and culture of exudates, or serological tests.
2. Treat cutaneous anthrax with 2 million units of penicillin G every 6 hours until the edema subsides. Follow that with oral penicillin G 500 mg q.6h. for 7–10 days. Skin lesions should be cleaned and covered.
3. Treat inhalation and other forms of anthrax with 2 million units of penicillin G very 2 hours.

Prophylaxis

Vaccines are available for agriculture workers, veterinary personnel, and others with increased risk.

AORTIC ANEURYSM

1. Confirm diagnosis with ultrasound, CT scan with contrast, VDRL, sedimentation rate, aortography.
2. *Atherosclerotic aneurysm:*
   a. Greater than 5 cm: Surgery.
   b. Less than 4 cm: Follow with frequent ultrasound measurements until 5 cm or more or becomes symptomatic.
   c. Rupture: Immediate surgery.
3. *Syphilitic aneurysm:* Antibiotics and surgery.
4. *Dissecting aneurysm:*
   a. Proximal (ascending aorta): Control blood pressure with sodium nitroprusside infusion and beta blockers IV. Surgery when stable.
   b. Distal (beyond the left subclavian artery): Control blood pressure with sodium nitroprusside infusion and IV beta blockers. May be able to avoid surgery; but if there is continued pain, do not delay.

Prognosis

Five-year survival for aneurysms greater than 5 cm is less than 20%, without surgery.

AORTIC ANEURYSM

CONFIRM DIAGNOSIS WITH
ULTRASOUND, AORTOGRAPHY, CT SCAN WITH CONTRAST, VDRL

ATHEROSCLEROTIC

- GREATER THAN 5 cm DIAMETER
  - SURGERY
- LESS THAN 4 cm DIAMETER
  - FOLLOW WITH REPEAT ULTRASOUND PERIODICALLY

SYPHILITIC

ANTIBIOTICS, SURGERY

DISSECTING

- PROXIMAL
  - CONTROL BLOOD PRESSURE
    - SURGERY
    - DISSECTION STOPS
      - SURGERY MAY NOT BE NECESSARY
- DISTAL
  - CONTROL BLOOD PRESSURE
    - DISSECTION CONTINUES
      - SURGERY

APLASTIC ANEMIA

1. Confirm diagnosis by CBC and bone marrow aspiration or biopsy. Exclude other causes of pancytopenia.
2. *Mild aplastic anemia:* Treat with supportive care including removal of all possible causes and immediate use of antibiotics for established infections. Prophylactic antibiotics should not be used. Transfusions should only be used in emergency situations.
3. *Moderate aplastic anemia:* In this stage, transfusions may be used judiciously for severe anemia, leukopenia, or bleeding. Platelet transfusions are the replacement fluid of choice in serious hemorrhage. These should be HLA compatible when possible. Marrow stimulation androgens and immunosuppressant agents may be useful at this stage. Consult a hematologist for guidance.
4. *Advanced aplastic anemia:* Bone marrow transplantation is indicated at this stage of the disease. The patient must be prepared with immunosuppressants and corticosteroids. They should be under the care of a hematologist experienced in this procedure.

ASCARIS LUMBRICOIDES

1. Confirm the diagnosis with stools for ovum and parasites and eosinophil counts.
2. Treat with mebendazole 100 mg p.o. b.i.d. for 3 days.
3. Alternatively, pyrantel pamoate 11 mg/kg may be given as a single dose (maximum of 1 g).

ASTHMA

1. Confirm diagnosis by pulmonary function tests before and after a beta-adrenergic agonist (epinephrine or isoproterenol). Sputum smear for eosinophils and skin tests may be helpful.
2. *Acute attacks:*
   a. Treat initially with oxygen and aerosolized albuterol or metaproterenol every 20 minutes by a hand-held nebulizer. Draw arterial blood gases.
   b. If this is ineffective and the patient is not hypertensive, administer terbutaline or epinephrine subcutaneously 0.1–0.3 cc.
   c. If the above are ineffective, IV aminophylline drip and corticosteroids (dexamethasone 6–8 mg q.4h.) are given, and the patient is admitted to the hospital. If blood gases indicate significant hypoxia or hypercarbia, the patient is admitted to the intensive care unit and a pulmonologist is consulted.
   d. Tracheotomy or intubation may be required.
3. *Chronic asthma:*
   a. Treat initially with aerosolized albuterol, isoetharine, or metaproterenol.
   b. If that is ineffective, administer albuterol 2–4 mg q.i.d. orally.
   c. If the above is ineffective, add inhaled corticosteroid such as beclomethasone (Beclovent, Vanceril) or triamcinolone acetonide (Azmacort).
   d. If the above are ineffective when used alone or together, add long-acting theophylline agent (Theo-Dur, Slo-phyllin) 100–300 mg b.i.d. Cromolyn sodium may be added at this point.
3. When all else fails, consider short but intense courses of oral or IM corticosteroids (prednisone 60 mg/day and tapering over a 2-week period). Consult an allergist or pulmonologist.

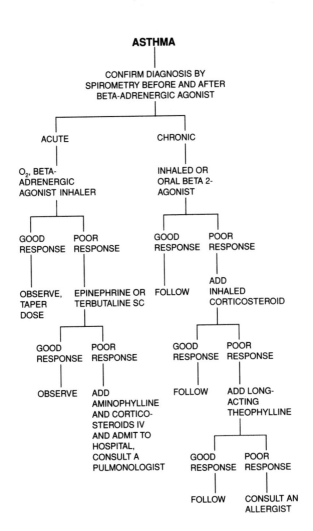

ASTHMA

CONFIRM DIAGNOSIS BY
SPIROMETRY BEFORE AND AFTER
BETA-ADRENERGIC AGONIST

ACUTE

O₂, BETA-
ADRENERGIC
AGONIST INHALER

GOOD
RESPONSE

OBSERVE,
TAPER
DOSE

POOR
RESPONSE

EPINEPHRINE OR
TERBUTALINE SC

GOOD
RESPONSE

OBSERVE

POOR
RESPONSE

ADD
AMINOPHYLLINE
AND CORTICO-
STEROIDS IV
AND ADMIT TO
HOSPITAL,
CONSULT A
PULMONOLOGIST

CHRONIC

INHALED OR
ORAL BETA 2-
AGONIST

GOOD
RESPONSE

FOLLOW

POOR
RESPONSE

ADD
INHALED
CORTICOSTEROID

GOOD
RESPONSE

FOLLOW

POOR
RESPONSE

ADD LONG-
ACTING
THEOPHYLLINE

GOOD
RESPONSE

FOLLOW

POOR
RESPONSE

CONSULT AN
ALLERGIST

Asthma   27

BALANTIDIASIS

1. Confirm diagnosis by stool for ovum and parasites.
2. Treat with tetracycline 500 mg q.i.d. for 10 days or with metronidazole 750 mg t.i.d. for 5 days.

BASILAR ARTERY INSUFFICIENCY OR THROMBOSIS

1. Confirm diagnosis by CT scanning to rule out hemorrhage, MRI angiography, or four-vessel selective radiocontrast angiography. Consult a neurologist and a radiologist.
2. Provided there is no significant hypertension, treat initially with heparin 5000–10,000 unit loading dose IV, following with 1000–1500 units IV hourly, based on PTT levels. If there is hypertension, antiplatelet therapy and antihypertensive therapy may be best.
3. Follow up with sodium warfarin orally for 6–12 months or longer if there are repeated attacks.
4. For occlusive disease of the branches of the basilar or vertebral artery, antiplatelet therapy may be sufficient. Consult a neurologist for guidance.

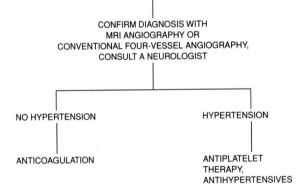

BASILAR ARTERY INSUFFICIENCY OR THROMBOSIS

CONFIRM DIAGNOSIS WITH
MRI ANGIOGRAPHY OR
CONVENTIONAL FOUR-VESSEL ANGIOGRAPHY,
CONSULT A NEUROLOGIST

NO HYPERTENSION   HYPERTENSION

ANTICOAGULATION   ANTIPLATELET
                         THERAPY,
                         ANTIHYPERTENSIVES

BELL'S PALSY

1. Confirm diagnosis by clinical picture, audiogram, x-rays of mastoids and petrous bones, and EMG in selected cases. When in doubt, consult a neurologist.
2. Treat with prednisone 60 mg/day for 1–3 weeks and gradually taper. In addition, administer acyclovir 200 mg five times a day for 10 days.
3. Alternatively, ACTH gel may be given IM 80 units a day for 3 days, 40 units a day for 3 days, 20 units a day for 3 days, and 10 units a day for 2 days.
4. Keep eyes moist with artificial tears, eye patch, and, in some cases, tarsorrhaphy. Consult an ophthalmologist.
5. If recovery is prolonged, begin physiotherapy (electrical stimulation, etc.). Consider referral to an otolaryngologist or a neurosurgeon.

BERIBERI

1. Confirm diagnosis with blood thiamine, pyruvate, urinary methylglyoxal, and erythrocyte transketolase activity.
2. Treat with 50–100 mg of thiamine IV or IM daily for 3–4 days and then 10 mg daily.
3. The patient should also receive multiple vitamins and a nutritious diet.
4. Treat congestive heart failure with digitalis and diuretics.
5. Look for alcoholism and treat.

BILIARY CIRRHOSIS

1. Confirm diagnosis with serum antimitochron-drial antibody titer and liver biopsy.
2. No specific therapy is available.
3. Colchicine may slow the progression of the disease.
4. Cholestyramine 8–12 g/day may relieve itching.
5. Treat steatorrhea with a low-fat diet.
6. Administer fat-soluble vitamin A and K to prevent blindness and bleeding.
7. Administer calcium and vitamin D to prevent osteoporosis.

BLASTOMYCOSIS

1. Confirm diagnosis with cultures of sputum, exudates, or urine.
2. Treat with amphotericin B over an 8- to 10-week period with a total dose of 2 g.
3. In patients with cavitary lung disease, the treatment should be extended to 12 weeks for a total dose of 2.5 g or more.
4. Alternatively, ketoconazole 400 mg/day can be used. If improvement is not noted after 1 month, the dose can be increased to 600–800 mg/day. Treatment should be continued for 6–12 months.

Administration of Amphotericin B

1. This drug must be given very carefully because reactions are common. An infectious disease expert should be consulted.
2. First a test dose of 1 mg in 20 ml of 5% dextrose is given IV.
3. If this is tolerated, a dose of 0.3 mg/kg is given in 50 cc of 5% dextrose solution over a 6-hour period on the first day of therapy.
4. After that, dose may be increased to 1 mg/kg daily, administered over a 6-hour period at 10 mg/100 ml of 5% dextrose and water.
5. Do not give any other drug in the same IV, and observe carefully for seizures, vomiting, and other drug reactions.

BORNHOLM'S DISEASE

1. Confirm diagnosis by viral isolation from throat, stool, and so on. Serologic tests may also be useful.
2. Treatment is symptomatic because there is no specific therapy.

BOTULISM

1. Confirm diagnosis by demonstration of toxin in the patient's serum, utilizing mice for a bioassay. Toxin may also be demonstrated in the vomitus or stool.
2. Treatment of food poisoning includes hospitalization, intensive care, respiratory support including intubation, removal of toxins from the GI tract with laxatives and emetics, and administering equine antitoxin.
3. Obtain antitoxin from the CDC by calling 1−404−639−3311 days and 1−404−329−3644 nights.
4. In wound botulism, administer an antibiotic such as penicillin, débride the wound, and administer equine antitoxin.
5. *Prognosis:* Mortality has dropped to 7.5% with modern therapy.

BRACHIAL PLEXUS NEUROPATHY

1. Confirm diagnosis by history, electromyography, nerve conduction velocity studies, and somatosensory evoked potentials. Consult a neurologist or a neurosurgeon.
2. Treatment is usually symptomatic with rest, immobilization, and proper nutrition. High-dose multiple B vitamins may be beneficial. Physiotherapy is important once the acute stage has passed. Consult a physiatrist.

BRAIN TUMORS, SELECTED

1. Confirm diagnosis with MRI or CT scans. Consult neurosurgeon.
2. Treat benign tumors such as meningiomas, acoustic neuromas, dermoid tumors, pituitary adenomas, and colloid cysts primarily by surgical resection. Malignant meningiomas and those which are incompletely removed may require radiation. Pituitary adenomas may be treated by radiation (see page 364).
3. Treat malignant tumors such as glioblastomas, ependymomas, medulloblastomas, and lymphoma by combined surgery, radiation, and chemotherapy. Consult an oncologist for guidance. Solitary metastatic tumors of the brain may be removed surgically in selected cases.

BRAIN TUMORS, SELECTED

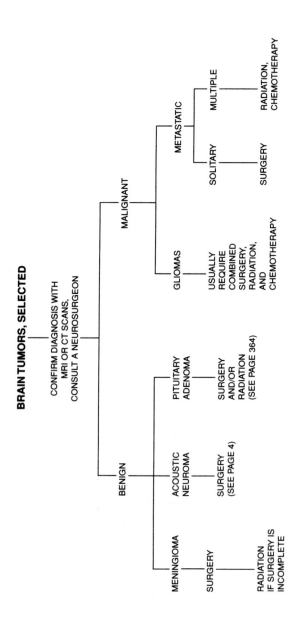

CONFIRM DIAGNOSIS WITH
MRI OR CT SCANS,
CONSULT A NEUROSURGEON

BENIGN

MENINGIOMA

SURGERY

RADIATION
IF SURGERY IS
INCOMPLETE

ACOUSTIC
NEUROMA

SURGERY
(SEE PAGE 4)

PITUITARY
ADENOMA

SURGERY
AND/OR
RADIATION
(SEE PAGE 364)

MALIGNANT

GLIOMAS

USUALLY
REQUIRE
COMBINED
SURGERY,
RADIATION,
AND
CHEMOTHERAPY

METASTATIC

SOLITARY

SURGERY

MULTIPLE

RADIATION,
CHEMOTHERAPY

BRONCHIAL ADENOMA

1. Confirm diagnosis by bronchoscopy and biopsy.
2. Treat with surgical resection. Consult a thoracic surgeon.

BRONCHIECTASIS

1. Confirm diagnosis with CT scan, bronchoscopy, bronchography, and sputum analysis.
2. Treat medically with postural drainage, bronchodilators, and antibiotics for acute exacerbations. Mucolytic agents are controversial.
3. Treat surgically with excision or embolization for local disease or massive hemorrhage.

BRONCHITIS, ACUTE

1. Confirm diagnosis with chest x-ray, sputum smear, and culture.
2. Initial treatment includes humidification, hydration, antipyretics, and anti-inflammatory agents because most cases are viral. Expectorants are of doubtful value.
3. If sputum cultures confirm a bacterial cause or patient's condition is critical, antibiotics should be given. Amoxicillin 500 mg t.i.d. for 10 days is suggested until culture and sensitivity studies are available. Alternatively, erythromycin 500 mg q.i.d. may be given.
4. Look for atypical pneumonia (page 370).
5. Antitussive agents should not be given if cough is productive.

BRUCELLOSIS

1. Confirm diagnosis by serological tests.
2. *Uncomplicated:*
   a. Treat with doxycycline 100 mg q.12h. and streptomycin 15 mg/kg q.12h. IM for 2 weeks.
   b. Alternatively, rifampin may be given instead of the streptomycin (15 mg/kg for 2 weeks). Also, trimethoprim-sulfamethoxazole (160 mg/800 mg) b.i.d. may be used.
3. *Complicated:*
   a. Endocarditis: Antibiotics and valve replacement.
   b. Abscess: Antibiotics plus surgical drainage.
   c. Neurobrucellosis: Doxycycline 100 mg q.12h and rifampin 10–15 mg/kg daily are the drugs of choice. They should be continued for 3–6 months.

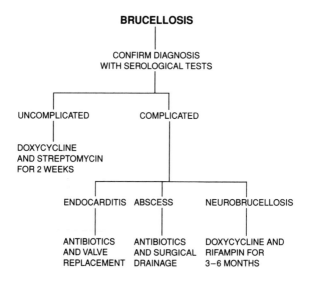

BRUCELLOSIS

CONFIRM DIAGNOSIS
WITH SEROLOGICAL TESTS

UNCOMPLICATED   COMPLICATED

DOXYCYCLINE
AND STREPTOMYCIN
FOR 2 WEEKS

ENDOCARDITIS   ABSCESS   NEUROBRUCELLOSIS

ANTIBIOTICS   ANTIBIOTICS   DOXYCYCLINE AND
AND VALVE   AND SURGICAL   RIFAMPIN FOR
REPLACEMENT   DRAINAGE   3–6 MONTHS

BURSITIS

1. Diagnosis is by clinical picture. Occasionally, fluid can be aspirated from the bursa, confirming the diagnosis. X-rays may show calcium deposits.
2. Treat with a mixture of 2–4 cc of 1.5% Xylocaine and 0.5–1.0 cc of triamcinolone diacetate (20–40 mg) injected into the bursa. This may be repeated once a week for three injections, if necessary. If pain persists after that, the diagnosis should be questioned or other modalities should be tried.
3. Conservative treatment includes NSAIDs and physiotherapy.
4. In persistent cases and patients with underlying disease (AIDS, diabetes mellitus), look for septic bursitis and treat with antibiotics.

CANCER OF THE STOMACH

1. Confirm diagnosis with gastroscopy and biopsy or exploratory laparotomy. Look for metastasis.
2. *Adenocarcinoma with no obvious metastasis:* Treat with surgery.
3. *Adenocarcinoma with metastasis:* Treat with surgery to relieve obstruction and control bleeding and follow with radiation and chemotherapy. Consult an oncologist.
4. *Lymphoma:*
   a. Resectable: Treat with surgery and follow with postoperative radiation.
   b. Unresectable: Treat with radiation and chemotherapy. Consult an oncologist.
5. *Leiomyosarcoma:* Treat with surgery.
6. *Prognosis:*
   a. Adenocarcinoma: If it is resectable, there is a 20% 5-year survival. If it is not resectable, there is only a 5–10% 5-year survival.
   b. Lymphoma: Resectable cases have a 50% 5-year survival.
   c. Leiomyosarcoma: Curable in most cases.

CANCER OF THE STOMACH

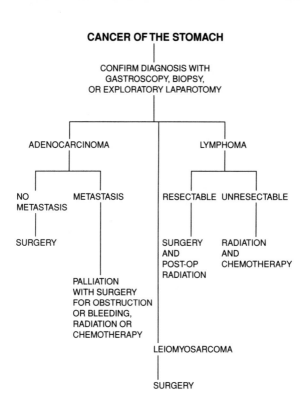

CONFIRM DIAGNOSIS WITH
GASTROSCOPY, BIOPSY,
OR EXPLORATORY LAPAROTOMY

ADENOCARCINOMA

LYMPHOMA

NO METASTASIS

METASTASIS

RESECTABLE   UNRESECTABLE

SURGERY

SURGERY
AND
POST-OP
RADIATION

RADIATION
AND
CHEMOTHERAPY

PALLIATION
WITH SURGERY
FOR OBSTRUCTION
OR BLEEDING,
RADIATION OR
CHEMOTHERAPY

LEIOMYOSARCOMA

SURGERY

CARBON MONOXIDE POISONING

1. Confirm diagnosis by blood carboxyhemoglobin level.
2. Treat mild to moderate cases with removal from contaminated area and 100% oxygen until CO level is 15.5% or less.
3. Treat severe cases with hyperbaric oxygen chamber. Call a poison control center to locate the chamber and transfer the patient.
4. If patient has a pH below 7.1, correct acidosis with sodium bicarbonate.
5. Pregnant patients must have oxygen continued for several hours. Consult an obstetrician.

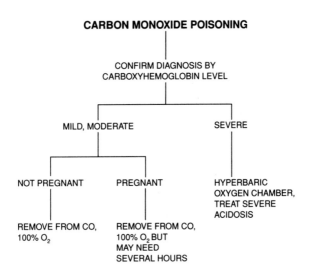

CARBON MONOXIDE POISONING

CONFIRM DIAGNOSIS BY CARBOXYHEMOGLOBIN LEVEL

MILD, MODERATE — SEVERE

NOT PREGNANT — PREGNANT

REMOVE FROM CO, 100% O_2

REMOVE FROM CO, 100% O_2 BUT MAY NEED SEVERAL HOURS

HYPERBARIC OXYGEN CHAMBER, TREAT SEVERE ACIDOSIS

CARBON TETRACHLORIDE POISONING

1. Confirm diagnosis by history and physical. Consult a poison control center.
2. Treat with prompt gastric lavage, but do not induce emesis or administer activated charcoal.
3. Administer oxygen and maintain respiratory, renal, liver, and cardiac function.
4. Monitor liver function tests.

CARBUNCLES AND FURUNCLES

1. Confirm diagnosis by clinical picture, smear, and culture of exudates.
2. Treat with warm saline soaks, antibiotics, and incision and drainage.
3. Carbuncles are often invasive, so excision is often necessary. If this is unsuccessful the first time, it must be repeated until all the sinus tracts are removed. Consult a general surgeon.

CARCINOID SYNDROME

1. Confirm diagnosis by measuring urinary 5-HIAA.
2. Resection of the primary tumor is rarely curative since almost all patients have metastasis at the time of diagnosis.
3. Treatment is primarily symptomatic:
   a. Diarrhea may be treated with cyproheptadine and methysergide.
   b. Flushing may be treated with an H-1 and H-2 antagonist such as diphenhydramine and ranitidine.
   c. Dyspnea and wheezing can be treated with theophylline and corticosteroids.
   d. Octreotide is a potent inhibitor of serotonin secretion and will reduce diarrhea and flushing.
4. Chemotherapy is available. Consult an oncologist.
5. *Prognosis:* The 5-year survival is 18% with liver metastasis.

CARCINOMA OF THE AMPULLA OF VATER

1. Confirm diagnosis with ERCP. Consult a gastroenterologist.
2. Treat with wide or radical excision of the tumor or a Whipple procedure.
3. *Prognosis:* The 5-year survival for tumors without metastasis approaches 40%.

CARCINOMA OF THE BREAST

1. Confirm diagnosis by mammography, fine needle aspiration, and needle or open biopsy. Decide on treatment with the help of an oncologist, a breast surgeon, and a radiotherapist.
2. *Tumors localized to breast without metastasis:*
   a. If the patient is concerned about cosmetics, limited surgery is done to remove the mass and limited node dissection, followed by breast conserving radiotherapy.
   b. If patient is unconcerned about cosmetic appearance, a simple mastectomy is done with node dissection, if necessary.
   c. Patients with a large mass will have to have a simple mastectomy, regardless.
3. *Tumors associated with lymph node metastasis:* Lumpectomy or mastectomy plus:
   a. Premenopausal patients: Most patients should receive adjuvant chemotherapy (such as cyclophosphamide plus doxorubicin). Consult an oncologist.
   b. Postmenopausal patients: Treat with tamoxifen for 2–5 years if receptor positive. Consult an oncologist.
4. Tumors with distant metastasis:
   a. With positive estrogen or progesterone receptor, treat with tamoxifen if postmenopausal and either tamoxifen or oophorectomy if premenopausal. Consult an oncologist.
   b. If there are no estrogen or progesterone receptors, then chemotherapy is prescribed. Consult an oncologist.
5. Breast reconstruction can be done at the time of simple mastectomy or later.

CARCINOMA OF THE BREAST

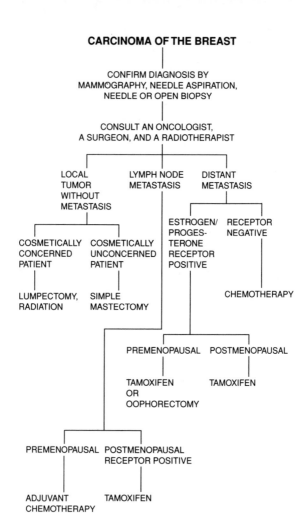

CONFIRM DIAGNOSIS BY
MAMMOGRAPHY, NEEDLE ASPIRATION,
NEEDLE OR OPEN BIOPSY

CONSULT AN ONCOLOGIST,
A SURGEON, AND A RADIOTHERAPIST

LOCAL TUMOR WITHOUT METASTASIS

LYMPH NODE METASTASIS

DISTANT METASTASIS

COSMETICALLY CONCERNED PATIENT

COSMETICALLY UNCONCERNED PATIENT

ESTROGEN/PROGESTERONE RECEPTOR POSITIVE

RECEPTOR NEGATIVE

LUMPECTOMY, RADIATION

SIMPLE MASTECTOMY

CHEMOTHERAPY

PREMENOPAUSAL

POSTMENOPAUSAL

TAMOXIFEN OR OOPHORECTOMY

TAMOXIFEN

PREMENOPAUSAL

POSTMENOPAUSAL RECEPTOR POSITIVE

ADJUVANT CHEMOTHERAPY

TAMOXIFEN

CARCINOMA OF THE CERVIX

1. Confirm diagnosis by colposcopy, Schiller test, and biopsy.
2. *Carcinoma in situ:* Treat with local cauterization, cryotherapy, cone biopsy, or hysterectomy.
3. *Invasive carcinoma:* Treat with irradiation in consultation with a radiotherapist and gynecologist. Radical hysterectomy may be indicated in some cases.
4. *Recurrent or persistent carcinoma:* Treat with pelvic exenteration.

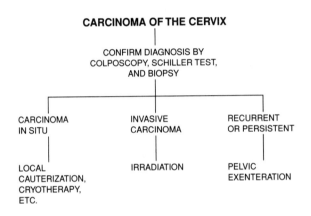

CARCINOMA OF THE CERVIX

CONFIRM DIAGNOSIS BY COLPOSCOPY, SCHILLER TEST, AND BIOPSY

CARCINOMA IN SITU — LOCAL CAUTERIZATION, CRYOTHERAPY, ETC.

INVASIVE CARCINOMA — IRRADIATION

RECURRENT OR PERSISTENT — PELVIC EXENTERATION

CARCINOMA OF THE COLON

1. Confirm diagnosis by colonoscopy and biopsy. Perform CEA, liver function tests, and CT scans to determine metastasis. Consult an abdominal surgeon.
2. Treat all tumors with resection, even if metastases are found.
3. Look for metastases before and during surgery.
4. Postoperative radiotherapy is given to patients with Duke's B or C tumors, especially if they penetrate the serosa.
5. Preoperative radiation of large fixed tumors may facilitate surgical removal.
6. Prophylactic chemotherapy after resection of Duke's B and C tumors is probably of no value.
7. Chemotherapy of advanced tumors is of limited value.
8. Follow with frequent CEA determinations.
9. *Prognosis:* This is better than 90% for tumors limited to the mucosa and submucosa. It is only 5% with patients who have distant metastasis.

CARCINOMA OF THE ENDOMETRIUM

1. Confirm diagnosis with Pap smears and endometrial biopsy.
2. No metastasis is evident preoperatively: Treat with total abdominal hysterectomy and bilateral salpingo-oophorectomy.
3. Follow surgery with postoperative irradiation if positive lymph nodes are found.
4. When distant metastasis is evident preoperatively or postoperatively, consult an oncologist for chemotherapy.

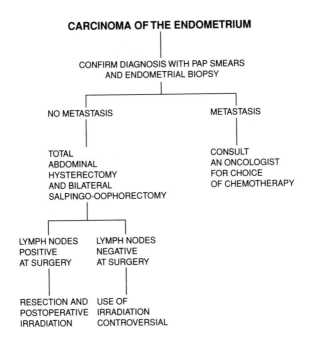

CARCINOMA OF THE LUNG

1. Confirm diagnosis by bronchoscopy and biopsy, needle biopsy, or open resection.
2. *Non-small-cell carcinoma:*
   a. Well-localized: Surgery. Consult a radiotherapist and an oncologist for radiation and/or chemotherapy.
   b. Not well localized.
3. *Small-cell carcinoma:*
   a. With limited spread: Treat with radiation and/or chemotherapy. Surgery may be done for staging purposes.
   b. Extensive: Treat with chemotherapy. Consult an oncologist.
4. *Treatment of complications:*
   a. Bronchial obstruction: Treat with laser obliteration of tumor through bronchoscope.
   b. Painful isolated metastasis: Treat with irradiation.
   c. Hypercalcemia: Treat with hydration, diphosphonates, steroids, and mithramycin.
   d. Superior vena cava obstruction: Irradiation.

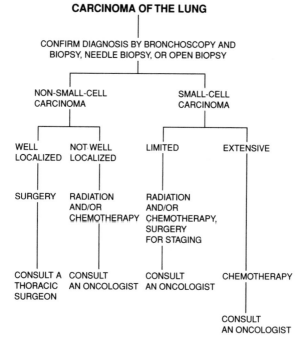

CARCINOMA OF THE OVARY

1. Confirm diagnosis by ultrasonography, laparoscopy, serum CA-125 levels, and exploratory laparotomy. Consult a gynecologist and an oncologist.
2. *Stage I and II:* Treat with total abdominal hysterectomy (TAH) and bilateral salpingo-oophorectomy (BSO) and surgical staging with careful follow-up. Some premenopausal women are eligible for unilateral salpingo-oophorectomy to preserve reproduction.
3. *Stage III and IV:* Treat with TAH and BSO, omentectomy, cytoreduction, and chemotherapy. In advanced cases, chemotherapy should continue for 3–6 months. After that, a second-look exploratory laparotomy should be done, and if residual tumor is found, additional chemotherapy is given.

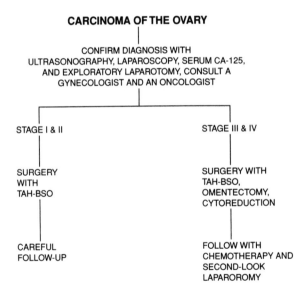

CARCINOMA OF THE OVARY

CONFIRM DIAGNOSIS WITH
ULTRASONOGRAPHY, LAPAROSCOPY, SERUM CA-125,
AND EXPLORATORY LAPAROTOMY, CONSULT A
GYNECOLOGIST AND AN ONCOLOGIST

STAGE I & II

SURGERY
WITH
TAH-BSO

CAREFUL
FOLLOW-UP

STAGE III & IV

SURGERY WITH
TAH-BSO,
OMENTECTOMY,
CYTOREDUCTION

FOLLOW WITH
CHEMOTHERAPY AND
SECOND-LOOK
LAPAROROMY

CARCINOMA OF THE PANCREAS

1. Confirm diagnosis with CT scan, ERCP, or exploratory laparotomy.
2. Determine resectability with chest films, CT scans, and celiac angiography.
3. *Resectable:* Consult a surgeon for Whipple procedure, intraoperative radiation, followed by chemotherapy.
4. *Nonresectable:* Consult an oncologist for consideration of external beam radiotherapy, 5-fluorouracil therapy, and other chemotherapy.
5. *Complications:* Treat biliary obstruction with palliative surgery, endoscopic stent placement, or transhepatic stent placement.
6. *Prognosis:* If the tumor is resectable, 3% are curable. If the tumor is unresectable, there is a 5-month median survival.

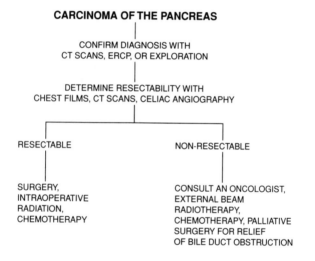

CARCINOMA OF THE PANCREAS
|
CONFIRM DIAGNOSIS WITH
CT SCANS, ERCP, OR EXPLORATION
|
DETERMINE RESECTABILITY WITH
CHEST FILMS, CT SCANS, CELIAC ANGIOGRAPHY

RESECTABLE   NON-RESECTABLE

SURGERY,   CONSULT AN ONCOLOGIST,
INTRAOPERATIVE   EXTERNAL BEAM
RADIATION,   RADIOTHERAPY,
CHEMOTHERAPY   CHEMOTHERAPY, PALLIATIVE
                              SURGERY FOR RELIEF
                              OF BILE DUCT OBSTRUCTION

CARDIAC ARREST

1. Confirm diagnosis by clinical assessment and EKG. Consult a cardiologist, if possible.
2. Begin CPR immediately. Draw arterial blood gases as soon as possible.
3. *Ventricular fibrillation:*
   a. Immediate defibrillation.
   b. Intubation and give O_2.
   c. If initial attempts at defibrillation fail, give bolus of 1 mg/kg of lidocaine IV and repeat defibrillation. Repeat lidocaine in 2 minutes and follow with continuous infusion of lidocaine 1–4 mg/min.
   d. Try intravenous procainamide 100/mg every 5 minutes, up to 500–800 mg, or bretylium tosylate 5–10 mg/kg in 5 minutes. Follow with maintenance dose.
   e. Epinephrine 0.5–1.0 mg IV or intracardiac may be tried every 5 minutes, also, while continuing defibrillation.
   f. Treat persistent acidosis with IV sodium bicarbonate 1 mmol/kg.
4. *Ventricular asystole or bradyarrhythmia:*
   a. Intubation and give O_2.
   b. Continue CPR.
   c. Epinephrine 0.5–1.0 mg IV or intracardiac.
   d. Atropine gr 1/150 may be tried.
5. *Postresuscitation care:* Consult a cardiologist.

CARDIAC ARREST

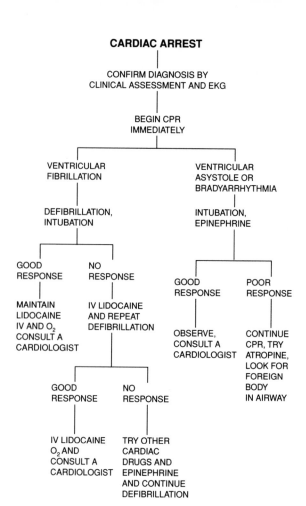

CONFIRM DIAGNOSIS BY
CLINICAL ASSESSMENT AND EKG

BEGIN CPR
IMMEDIATELY

VENTRICULAR
FIBRILLATION

VENTRICULAR
ASYSTOLE OR
BRADYARRHYTHMIA

DEFIBRILLATION,
INTUBATION

INTUBATION,
EPINEPHRINE

GOOD
RESPONSE

NO
RESPONSE

GOOD
RESPONSE

POOR
RESPONSE

MAINTAIN
LIDOCAINE
IV AND O₂
CONSULT A
CARDIOLOGIST

IV LIDOCAINE
AND REPEAT
DEFIBRILLATION

OBSERVE,
CONSULT A
CARDIOLOGIST

CONTINUE
CPR, TRY
ATROPINE,
LOOK FOR
FOREIGN
BODY
IN AIRWAY

GOOD
RESPONSE

NO
RESPONSE

IV LIDOCAINE
O₂ AND
CONSULT A
CARDIOLOGIST

TRY OTHER
CARDIAC
DRUGS AND
EPINEPHRINE
AND CONTINUE
DEFIBRILLATION

CARDIAC ARRHYTHMIAS

1. Confirm diagnosis by EKG, Holter monitoring, His bundle recording, and electrophysiologic assessment. Consult a cardiologist.
2. *Bradyarrhythmias:*
   a. Sinus node dysfunction: Treatment usually involves a permanent pacemaker.
   b. Fist-degree heart block: Usually no treatment is necessary.
   c. Second- and third-degree heart block: If the condition is felt to be due to drug toxicity, withdraw the drug and insert a temporary pacemaker. if there is persistent block, then a permanent pacemaker is utilized.
   d. Ventricular asystole: See Cardiac Arrest, page 59.
3. *Tachyarrhythmias:*
   a. APCs: No treatment is necessary unless symptomatic. Alcohol, tobacco, and caffeine should be withdrawn. A beta blocker may be tried; otherwise, consult a cardiologist.
   b. VPCs: No treatment is necessary if they are asymptomatic. If symptomatic, try a beta blocker first. If this is unsuccessful, quinidine may be utilized. In VPCs associated with myocardial infarction, the use of lidocaine, except in young patients, is controversial.
   c. Supraventricular tachycardia (SVT): If there is hypotension, treat with IV phenylephrine in 0.1 mg increments. If this is unsuccessful, verapamil 2.5–10 mg IV may be tried. Propanolol is also useful. If there is no hypotension, carotid sinus massage may terminate the attack. Temporary pacing may be necessary.
   d. Atrial flutter: Treat with cardioversion, followed by quinidine, flecainide, or amiodarone to prevent recurrences.
   e. Atrial fibrillation: Look for a possible cause such as thyrotoxicosis, alcoholic intoxication, and so on. Treat with digitalis or beta blockers. Medical or electrical cardioversion may be necessary. Consult a cardiologist.
   f. Ventricular tachycardia: If there is significant organic heart disease, immediate cardiover-

sion is indicated. If not, a cardiologist should be consulted for guidance.

g. Ventricular fibrillation: See Cardiac Arrest, page 59.

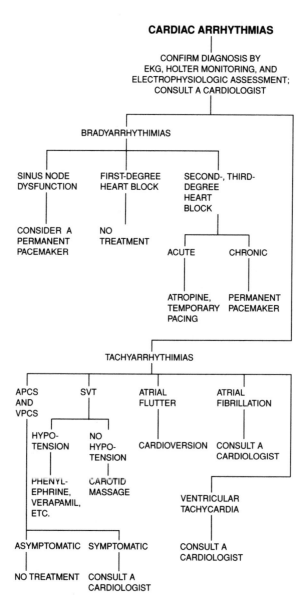

CARDIAC ARRHYTHMIAS

CONFIRM DIAGNOSIS BY
EKG, HOLTER MONITORING, AND
ELECTROPHYSIOLOGIC ASSESSMENT;
CONSULT A CARDIOLOGIST

BRADYARRHYTHIMIAS

- SINUS NODE DYSFUNCTION → CONSIDER A PERMANENT PACEMAKER
- FIRST-DEGREE HEART BLOCK → NO TREATMENT
- SECOND-, THIRD-DEGREE HEART BLOCK
  - ACUTE → ATROPINE, TEMPORARY PACING
  - CHRONIC → PERMANENT PACEMAKER

TACHYARRHYTHIMIAS

- APCS AND VPCS
  - ASYMPTOMATIC → NO TREATMENT
  - SYMPTOMATIC → CONSULT A CARDIOLOGIST
- SVT
  - HYPOTENSION → PHENYLEPHRINE, VERAPAMIL, ETC.
  - NO HYPOTENSION → CAROTID MASSAGE
- ATRIAL FLUTTER → CARDIOVERSION
- ATRIAL FIBRILLATION → CONSULT A CARDIOLOGIST
- VENTRICULAR TACHYCARDIA → CONSULT A CARDIOLOGIST

CARDIOMYOPATHY

1. Confirm diagnosis with cardiology consult, EKG, echocardiography, cardiac catheterization and myocardial biopsy. Consult a cardiologist.
2. *Congestive cardiomyopathy:* Treat as in congestive heart failure with diuretics occasionally, digoxin, and ACE inhibitors. If poor response, give vasodilators such as nitroglycerin, or hydralazine 25–75 mg t.i.d. Anticoagulants should be administered if CHF persists.
3. *Restrictive cardiomyopathy:* Medical therapy is disappointing, but corticosteroids may be used in sarcoid cardiomyopathy, deferoxamine and phlebotomy may be used in hemochromatosis, and surgery may be used for endomyocardial fibroelastosis.
4. *Hypertrophic cardiomyopathy:* Beta blockers, calcium channel blockers, and disopyramide should be tried. If poor response, consider dual chamber pacing and surgery.
5. *Complications:*
   a. When arrhythmias develop in hypertrophic cardiomyopathy, amiodarone may be useful, but avoid digoxin.
   b. Anticoagulants for embolization.
   c. When patient fails to respond to anything, cardiac transplant may be considered.

CARDIOMYOPATHY

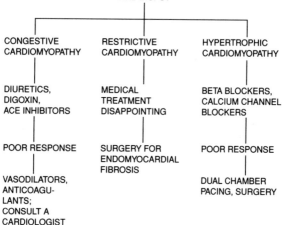

CONFIRM DIAGNOSIS WITH CARDIOLOGY CONSULT,
EKG, ECHOCARDIOGRAPHY, CARDIAC CATHETERIZATION,
AND BIOPSY

CONGESTIVE CARDIOMYOPATHY	RESTRICTIVE CARDIOMYOPATHY	HYPERTROPHIC CARDIOMYOPATHY
DIURETICS, DIGOXIN, ACE INHIBITORS	MEDICAL TREATMENT DISAPPOINTING	BETA BLOCKERS, CALCIUM CHANNEL BLOCKERS
POOR RESPONSE	SURGERY FOR ENDOMYOCARDIAL FIBROSIS	POOR RESPONSE
VASODILATORS, ANTICOAGULANTS; CONSULT A CARDIOLOGIST		DUAL CHAMBER PACING, SURGERY

CARPAL TUNNEL SYNDROME

1. Confirm diagnosis by referral to a neurologist for nerve conduction studies (NCV) of the median nerves.
2. Look for systemic causes such as rheumatoid arthritis, hypothyroidism, acromegaly, and so on.
3. *Mild disease and patient does not want surgery:*
   a. Treat with splints, NSAIDs, vitamin B_6.
   b. If poor response, try corticosteroid injections of carpal tunnel by an experienced physician.
   c. If poor response, refer to an orthopedic or neurological surgeon for surgery.
4. *Moderate to severe:* Refer to an orthopedic or neurological surgeon for surgery.
5. *Poor results from surgery:* Look for diabetes, alcoholism, and other causes of neuropathy.

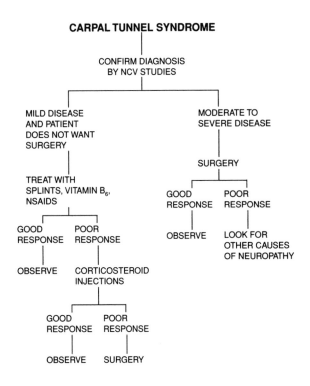

CAT-SCRATCH DISEASE

1. Confirm by lymph-node biopsy or clinical picture.
2. Treatment is symptomatic in most cases.
3. In immunocompromised patients (AIDS, etc.), bacillary angiomatosis may develop. Treat with erythromycin 500 mg q.i.d. p.o. or doxycycline 100 mg b.i.d. p.o. for 3 weeks.
4. If there is systemic spread, treat with aminoglycosides initially and follow with erythromycin or norfloxacin (400 mg b.i.d. p.o.).

CELLULITIS

1. Confirm diagnosis with smear and cultures of exudates.
2. Apply warm soaks and elevation (provided circulation is good).
3. Treat with oxacillin 1–2 g IV q.6h. for severe infections, and treat with dicloxacillin 500 mg p.o. q.6h. for mild to moderate infections.
4. Incision and drainage should be done once pus is well localized or if there is an inadequate response to antibiotics. Consult a surgeon.
5. Alternate antibiotics are cephalexin or erythromycin in penicillin-sensitive patients.
6. Consider hospitalization for patients with fever or other systemic reactions.
7. Look for underlying systemic disease (diabetes, etc.).

CEREBRAL ABSCESS

1. Confirm diagnosis by CT scans, MRI, or angiography.
2. Look for primary focus of infection (sinuses, etc.).
3. Culture of aspiration obtained by stereotactic CT guidance. Blood cultures are also helpful.
4. *Single small or multiple small abscesses:* Treat with IV aqueous penicillin G20–24 million units a day and metronidazole 750 mg t.i.d. Alternatively, chloramphenicol 1.0–1.5 g IV q.6h. may be given with the penicillin. Continue for 4–6 weeks. Follow progress with CT scans. If poor response, consult neurosurgeon for immediate surgery and continue antibiotics.
5. *Large abscesses:* Consult a neurosurgeon for immediate surgery and administer antibiotics both pre- and postoperatively.

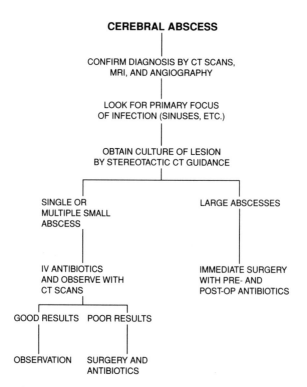

CEREBRAL ANEURYSM

1. Confirm diagnosis with cerebral angiography.
2. Confirm bleeding with CT scan and/or spinal tap. Consult a neurosurgeon.
3. *Unruptured:*
   a. Small: May observe until optimum time for surgery is established.
   b. Over 1 cm or producing signs of compression: Treat with immediate surgery.
4. *Ruptured:*
   a. Stable: Surgery may be postponed 1–2 weeks until optimum time is established.
   b. Unstable: Treat with antihypertensives and volume expanders until stable, then surgery.
   c. Patient remains unstable: Immediate surgery is the only hope for survival.
5. *Prognosis:* A large unruptured aneurysm has a 50% chance of rupture within 3 months. Once an aneurysm has ruptured, the mortality is 60% in 6 months if left untreated. Operative mortality is now down to 5% in medically stable patients.

CEREBRAL ANEURYSM

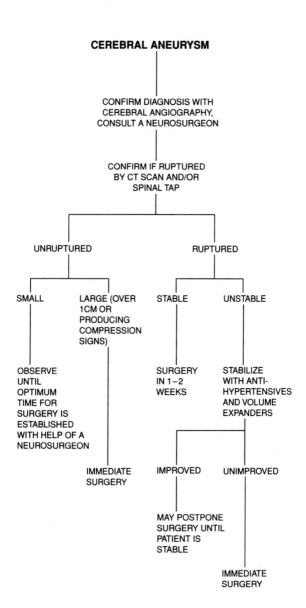

CONFIRM DIAGNOSIS WITH
CEREBRAL ANGIOGRAPHY,
CONSULT A NEUROSURGEON

CONFIRM IF RUPTURED
BY CT SCAN AND/OR
SPINAL TAP

UNRUPTURED

RUPTURED

SMALL

LARGE (OVER
1CM OR
PRODUCING
COMPRESSION
SIGNS)

STABLE

UNSTABLE

OBSERVE
UNTIL
OPTIMUM
TIME FOR
SURGERY IS
ESTABLISHED
WITH HELP OF A
NEUROSURGEON

SURGERY
IN 1–2
WEEKS

STABILIZE
WITH ANTI-
HYPERTENSIVES
AND VOLUME
EXPANDERS

IMMEDIATE
SURGERY

IMPROVED

UNIMPROVED

MAY POSTPONE
SURGERY UNTIL
PATIENT IS
STABLE

IMMEDIATE
SURGERY

CEREBRAL EMBOLISM

1. Confirm diagnosis with CT scans, MRI, and/or spinal tap.
2. Find embolic source.
3. Treat significant hypertension (see page 150).
4. *Severe neurologic deficit:*
   a. Acute stage: Do not use anticoagulants. Treat cerebral edema with osmotic solutions such as mannitol.
   b. After acute stage: Consider anticoagulants (sodium warfarin).
5. *Mild to moderate focal neurologic deficits:*
   a. Acute stage: Treat with heparin 5000–10,000 unit bolus, followed by 1000–1500 units IV per hour to maintain PTT at 1.5–2.5 times the control.
   b. After acute stage: Treat with sodium warfarin for 6–9 months to prevent further embolization.
6. Consult cardiovascular surgeon to treat emboli-producing lesions in the heart or carotid arteries.
7. Stroke rehabilitation.
8. *Prognosis:* Cerebral infarction in general is fatal in 20% of cases.

CEREBRAL EMBOLISM

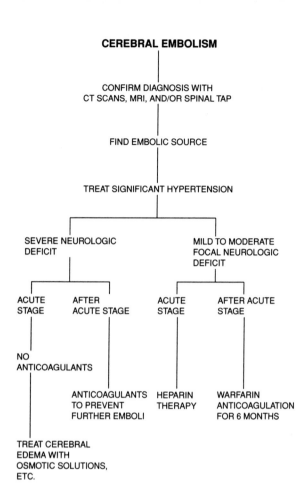

CONFIRM DIAGNOSIS WITH
CT SCANS, MRI, AND/OR SPINAL TAP

FIND EMBOLIC SOURCE

TREAT SIGNIFICANT HYPERTENSION

SEVERE NEUROLOGIC DEFICIT

MILD TO MODERATE FOCAL NEUROLOGIC DEFICIT

ACUTE STAGE

AFTER ACUTE STAGE

ACUTE STAGE

AFTER ACUTE STAGE

NO ANTICOAGULANTS

ANTICOAGULANTS TO PREVENT FURTHER EMBOLI

HEPARIN THERAPY

WARFARIN ANTICOAGULATION FOR 6 MONTHS

TREAT CEREBRAL EDEMA WITH OSMOTIC SOLUTIONS, ETC.

CEREBRAL THROMBOSIS AND INFARCTION

1. Confirm diagnosis with CT scan or MRI. Arteriography may be necessary. Consult a neurologist.
2. Look for hypercoagulable states or collagen disease.
3. *Thrombosis due to hypercoagulable state:* Treat with heparin, venesection, or chemotherapy. Consult an oncologist or a hematologist.
4. *Thrombosis with collagen disease:* Consult a rheumatologist. Treat specific disease.
5. *Thrombosis without hypercoagulable state or collagen disease:* Treat with supportive care and rehabilitation. Look for carotid or vertebral–basilar disease.
6. *Prognosis:* Mortality in cerebral infarcts is 20%.

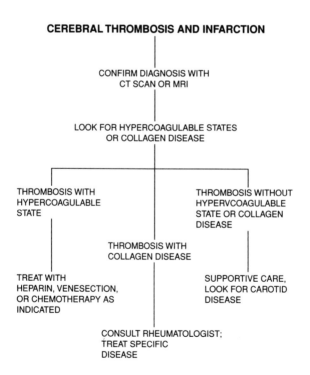

CEREBRAL THROMBOSIS AND INFARCTION

CONFIRM DIAGNOSIS WITH
CT SCAN OR MRI

LOOK FOR HYPERCOAGULABLE STATES
OR COLLAGEN DISEASE

THROMBOSIS WITH
HYPERCOAGULABLE
STATE

THROMBOSIS WITHOUT
HYPERVCOAGULABLE
STATE OR COLLAGEN
DISEASE

THROMBOSIS WITH
COLLAGEN DISEASE

TREAT WITH
HEPARIN, VENESECTION,
OR CHEMOTHERAPY AS
INDICATED

SUPPORTIVE CARE,
LOOK FOR CAROTID
DISEASE

CONSULT RHEUMATOLOGIST;
TREAT SPECIFIC
DISEASE

CERVICAL SPONDYLOSIS

1. Confirm diagnosis with x-rays, MRI, EMG, or evoked potential studies (DSEP). Consult a neurologist.
2. *No objectives neurologic findings:*
   a. Neck pain only: Treat with muscle relaxants, NSAIDs, cervical collar, physiotherapy.
   b. Radicular pain: Muscle relaxants, NSAIDs, cervical traction beginning at 8 lb and gradually increasing to as much as 12 lb to 20 lb in upright position. If that is ineffective, try nerve blocks with steroids and lidocaine. Consult a neurologist or an anesthesiologist. If that is ineffective, consider surgery.
3. *Objective neurologic findings:*
   a. Radiculopathy: Treat with cervical traction and nerve blocks. If that is ineffective, consult neurosurgeon for laminectomy or anterior body fusion.
   b. Myelopathy: Treat with laminectomy. Consult a neurosurgeon.

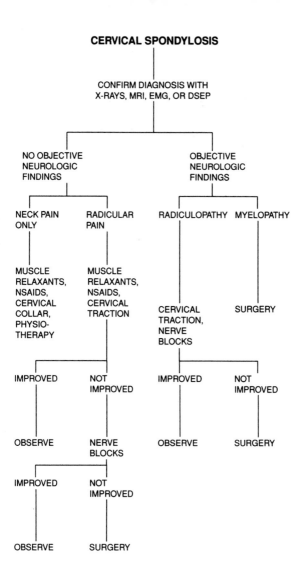

CERVICAL SPONDYLOSIS

CONFIRM DIAGNOSIS WITH
X-RAYS, MRI, EMG, OR DSEP

NO OBJECTIVE
NEUROLOGIC
FINDINGS

OBJECTIVE
NEUROLOGIC
FINDINGS

NECK PAIN
ONLY

RADICULAR
PAIN

RADICULOPATHY   MYELOPATHY

MUSCLE
RELAXANTS,
NSAIDS,
CERVICAL
COLLAR,
PHYSIO-
THERAPY

MUSCLE
RELAXANTS,
NSAIDS,
CERVICAL
TRACTION

CERVICAL
TRACTION,
NERVE
BLOCKS

SURGERY

IMPROVED

NOT
IMPROVED

IMPROVED

NOT
IMPROVED

OBSERVE

NERVE
BLOCKS

OBSERVE

SURGERY

IMPROVED

NOT
IMPROVED

OBSERVE

SURGERY

CERVICITIS

1. Confirm diagnosis with smear and cultures and cervical biopsy. Carefully exclude carcinoma and sexually transmitted diseases.
2. Treat with doxycycline 100 mg b.i.d for 7 days.
3. Alternatively, erythromycin 500 mg q.i.d. may be given for 7 days.
4. Treat chronic cervicitis with cauterization, conization, or cryosurgery. Consult a gynecologist. Remember, cervicitis is an important cause of infertility.

CHANCROID

1. Confirm diagnosis with smears and cultures of lesion. Biopsy may be necessary.
2. Treat with erythromycin 500 mg q.i.d. orally for 7 days.
3. Alternatively, give ceftriaxone 250 mg IM as a single dose or trimethoprim/sulfamethoxazole (160 mg/800 mg) b.i.d. orally for 5–7 days.

CHOLANGIOCARCINOMA

1. Confirm diagnosis by IV cholangiography, percutaneous transhepatic cholangiography, CT scan, or ERCP. Consult a gastroenterologist.
2. Most of these tumors are inoperable at the time of discovery. Treatment is with radiation and/or chemotherapy.
3. *Prognosis:* This is uniformly poor.

CHOLANGITIS

1. Confirm diagnosis with liver function tests, CT scan, or ultrasound. ERCP or percutaneous transhepatic cholangiography may be done after infection is brought under control.
2. Begin IV fluids and IV antibiotics (ampicillin plus an aminoglycoside or a second- or third-generation cephalosporin); intubation.
3. If severely ill or in shock, surgery without delay. (Consult general surgeon.)
4. If not severely ill, delay surgery until afebrile for 48 hours.
5. *Prognosis:* Eighty percent of patients respond to antibiotics and subsequent surgery.

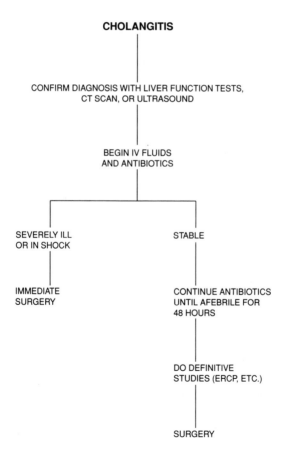

CHOLANGITIS

CONFIRM DIAGNOSIS WITH LIVER FUNCTION TESTS, CT SCAN, OR ULTRASOUND

BEGIN IV FLUIDS AND ANTIBIOTICS

SEVERELY ILL OR IN SHOCK

STABLE

IMMEDIATE SURGERY

CONTINUE ANTIBIOTICS UNTIL AFEBRILE FOR 48 HOURS

DO DEFINITIVE STUDIES (ERCP, ETC.)

SURGERY

CHOLECYSTITIS AND CHOLELITHIASIS

1. Confirm diagnosis by ultrasonography, oral cholecystography or radionuclide excretion scan (HIDA scan). Consult an abdominal surgeon.
2. *Acute:* Treat with hospitalization, nasogastric suction, IV fluids, antibiotics, and narcotics.
   a. Good response: Plan surgery after acute episode is over.
   b. Poor response: Immediate surgery.
3. *Chronic:*
   a. Asymptomatic: In patients with large stones (> 2 cm) or a calcified gallbladder, consider surgery. In patients with small stones (< 5 mm) consider a course of chenodiol or ursodiol. Diabetics should have a cholecystectomy regardless of the size of stones.
   b. Symptomatic: Treat with cholecystectomy.

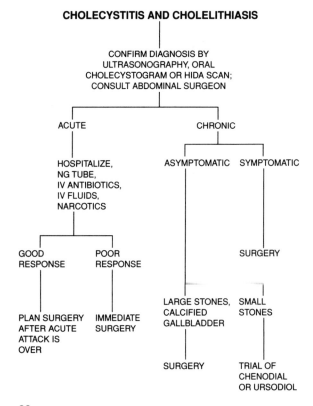

CHOLECYSTITIS AND CHOLELITHIASIS

CONFIRM DIAGNOSIS BY ULTRASONOGRAPHY, ORAL CHOLECYSTOGRAM OR HIDA SCAN; CONSULT ABDOMINAL SURGEON

ACUTE

HOSPITALIZE, NG TUBE, IV ANTIBIOTICS, IV FLUIDS, NARCOTICS

GOOD RESPONSE

POOR RESPONSE

PLAN SURGERY AFTER ACUTE ATTACK IS OVER

IMMEDIATE SURGERY

CHRONIC

ASYMPTOMATIC

SYMPTOMATIC

SURGERY

LARGE STONES, CALCIFIED GALLBLADDER

SMALL STONES

SURGERY

TRIAL OF CHENODIAL OR URSODIOL

CHOLEDOCHOLITHIASIS

1. Confirm diagnosis with ultrasonography, HIDA scanning, percutaneous transhepatic cholangiography (PTC), or endoscopic retrograde cholangiopancreatography (ERCP).
2. If septic, begin IV antibiotics.
3. If patient is stable, try to remove or dislodge the stone with ERCP or PTC. Consult a gastroenterologist.
4. If patient is unstable or acutely ill, perform cholecystectomy and/or common duct exploration. Consult a general surgeon.
5. *Prognosis:* Good for recovery in most cases.

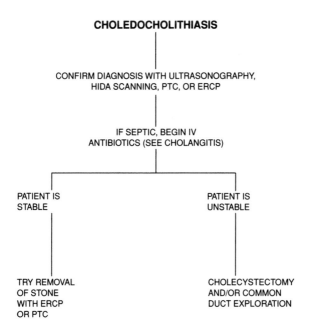

CHOLEDOCHOLITHIASIS

CONFIRM DIAGNOSIS WITH ULTRASONOGRAPHY,
HIDA SCANNING, PTC, OR ERCP

IF SEPTIC, BEGIN IV
ANTIBIOTICS (SEE CHOLANGITIS)

PATIENT IS STABLE

PATIENT IS UNSTABLE

TRY REMOVAL OF STONE WITH ERCP OR PTC

CHOLECYSTECTOMY AND/OR COMMON DUCT EXPLORATION

CHOLERA

1. Confirm diagnosis with stool smear and/or culture.
2. *Patient is severely ill or vomiting:* Catheterize the urinary bladder and run IV fluid in as rapidly as possible, wait until stable, and then give the rest of estimated fluid slowly. Keep a record of I&O.
3. *Patient is stable and not vomiting:* Use oral rehydration therapy with 3.5 g of salt, 1.5 g of potassium chloride, 2.5 g of sodium bicarbonate, and 20 g of glucose per 1000 cc of water.
4. Tetracycline or co-trimoxazole for 3 days. For IV administration dosage: Use Ringer's lactate, Hartman's solution, or Darrow's solution, but add adequate potassium.
5. *Prognosis:* Untreated cholera has a mortality of fifty percent. If properly treated there is a mortality of one percent or less.

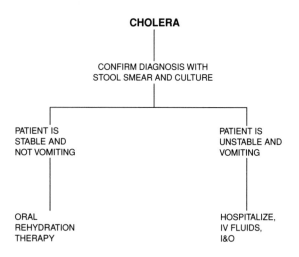

CHORIOCARCINOMA

1. Confirm diagnosis by elevated level of B subunit of hCG in plasma (pregnancy test). Consult an oncologist.
2. *In women:* Treat with dactinomycin and/or methotrexate.
3. *In men:* See Testicular Tumors.

CIRRHOSIS, ALCOHOLIC

1. Confirm diagnosis with liver function tests and biopsy.
2. *Uncomplicated:* Total abstinence from alcohol, high protein, high-calorie diet. Refer to Alcoholics Anonymous and psychotherapist.
3. *Complicated:*
   a. Liver failure: NPO, enemas to sterilize the bowel.
      - Neomycin 1 g q.6h. to sterilize bowel.
      - Consider hemodialysis: Consult nephrologist.
      - Cimetidine 200 mg q.8h. IV to keep acidity down.
      - IV dextrose with appropriate electrolytes.
      - Restrict protein intake.
      - Restrict drugs.
      - Consider liver transplant.
   b. Bleeding esophageal varices:
      - Confirm with endoscopy.
      - Type and cross 6 units of blood.
      - Vasopressin IV 20 units in 200 ml 5% D&W.
      - Pass Sengstaken–Blakemore tube.
      - Surgery if Sengstaken–Blakemore tube ineffective: Consult a general surgeon.
      - Portal–caval shunt later to reduce varices.
4. *Prognosis:* Twenty-five percent five-year survival. After bleeding esophageal varices only, 30–60% survive.

COCCIDIOMYCOSIS

1. Confirm diagnosis with chest x-ray, complement fixation titers, skin test.
2. *Mild to moderate primary pulmonary infection in patients with little risk:* Observe.
3. *Persistent primary pulmonary infections or infection in patients with increased risk (blacks, Asian, pregnant, immunocompromised):* Amphotericin B 1–3 g, depending on clinical response. See page 33 for technique of administration. Alternative drugs are ketoconazole 400 mg a day or itraconazole 200 mg b.i.d. Consult a pulmonologist.
4. *Chronic pulmonary disease with cavitation:* Surgical resection in addition to antifungal therapy indicated above.
5. *Bone disease:* Surgical débridement and amphotericin B, followed by ketoconazole or itraconazole for 9–12 months.
6. *Meningitis:* Intrathecal amphotericin B 0.5 mg three times a week.
7. *Disseminated disease:* Treat as bone disease.
8. Continue treatment until all evidence of the disease is gone, the complement fixation titers have diminished or stabilized, and cell-mediated immunity has been reestablished.

COCCIDIOMYCOSIS

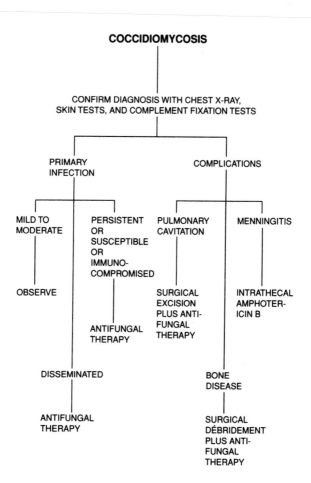

CONFIRM DIAGNOSIS WITH CHEST X-RAY,
SKIN TESTS, AND COMPLEMENT FIXATION TESTS

PRIMARY INFECTION

COMPLICATIONS

MILD TO MODERATE

PERSISTENT OR SUSCEPTIBLE OR IMMUNO-COMPROMISED

PULMONARY CAVITATION

MENNINGITIS

OBSERVE

ANTIFUNGAL THERAPY

SURGICAL EXCISION PLUS ANTI-FUNGAL THERAPY

INTRATHECAL AMPHOTER-ICIN B

DISSEMINATED

BONE DISEASE

ANTIFUNGAL THERAPY

SURGICAL DÉBRIDEMENT PLUS ANTI-FUNGAL THERAPY

CONJUNCTIVITIS

1. Confirm diagnosis with Gram's or Giemsa stained smears and cultures of eye exudate.
2. Exclude other causes of acute red eye, such as glaucoma, foreign body, keratitis, etc.
3. *Bacterial conjunctivitis:*
   a. Non-gonococcal: Treat with topical sulfacetamide ointment or drops 3–4 times daily for 5–7 days. Alternatively, bacitracin/polymyxin ointment or drops may be used. Do not use ointments or drops with neomycin. Oral antibiotics may facilitate recovery.
   b. Gonococcal: Consult ophthalmologist for IV or IM ceftriaxone therapy.
4. *Non-bacterial conjunctivitis:*
   a. Chlamydia: Treat with doxycycline 100 mg b.i.d. orally for ten days or erythromycin 40–50 mg/kg/day for three weeks.
   b. Viral conjunctivitis: Refer to ophthalmologist.
   c. Allergic conjunctivitis: Treat with antihistamines and corticosteroids topically and orally. For example, Decadron ophthalmic drops may be applied topically every two to four hours.

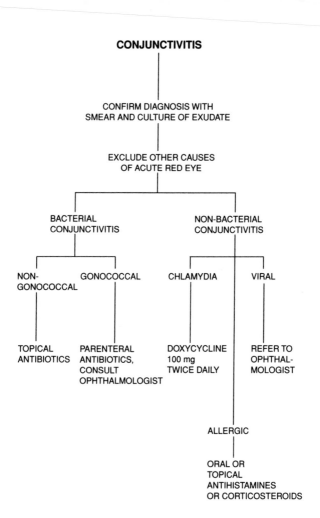

CONJUNCTIVITIS

CONFIRM DIAGNOSIS WITH
SMEAR AND CULTURE OF EXUDATE

EXCLUDE OTHER CAUSES
OF ACUTE RED EYE

BACTERIAL
CONJUNCTIVITIS

NON-BACTERIAL
CONJUNCTIVITIS

NON-
GONOCOCCAL

GONOCOCCAL

CHLAMYDIA

VIRAL

TOPICAL
ANTIBIOTICS

PARENTERAL
ANTIBIOTICS,
CONSULT
OPHTHALMOLOGIST

DOXYCYCLINE
100 mg
TWICE DAILY

REFER TO
OPHTHAL-
MOLOGIST

ALLERGIC

ORAL OR
TOPICAL
ANTIHISTAMINES
OR CORTICOSTEROIDS

CONGENITAL HEART DISEASE

1. Confirm diagnosis with EKG, echocardiography, chest x-ray, cardiac catheterization, and angio-cardiography.
2. *Atrial septal defect (ASD):*
   a. Small—observe; prophylactic antibiotics.
   b. Large with increased pulmonary flow—surgery.
   c. Surgery is contraindicated once significant pulmonary hypertension and shunt reversal have occurred.
3. *Ventricular septal defect (VSD):*
   a. Small—observe; prophylactic antibiotics as needed.
   b. Large—surgery.
   c. Infant with CHF: Treat with digitalis and diuretics; once stable, refer for surgery.
4. *Coarctation of the aorta:*
   a. Surgery in all but the mildest cases.
   b. Prophylactic antibiotics.
5. *Patent ductus arteriosus:*
   a. Spontaneous closure may occur.
   b. Try percutaneous occlusion with Rushkind umbrella.
   c. Conservative management in small shunts.
   d. Prophylactic antibiotics.
   e. Surgery when percutaneous occlusion unsuccessful.
6. *Pulmonic stenosis:*
   a. Mild: Observe.
   b. Larger with greater than 50-mm pressure drop across the pulmonic valve: Surgery.
   c. Prophylactic antibiotics.
7. *Tetralogy of Fallot:*
   a. Discovery in infancy: Perform Blalock shunt or Waterston shunt.
   b. After infancy: Surgery to repair pulmonic stenosis and ventricular septal defect.
   c. Prophylactic antibiotics.
8. *Transportation of great vessels:*
   a. Infancy: Balloon septostomy to create atrial septal defect.
   b. Later: Definitive surgery.
   c. Prophylactic antibiotics.

CONGENITAL HEART DISEASE

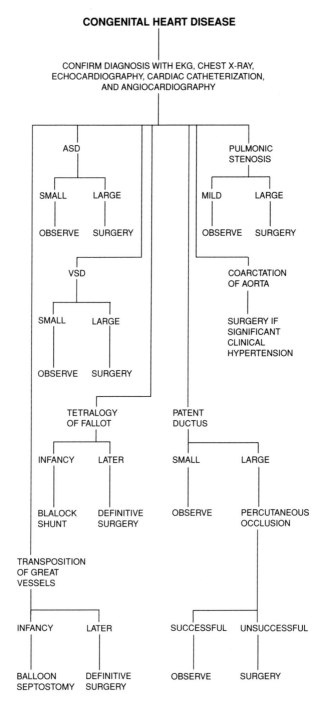

CONFIRM DIAGNOSIS WITH EKG, CHEST X-RAY, ECHOCARDIOGRAPHY, CARDIAC CATHETERIZATION, AND ANGIOCARDIOGRAPHY

ASD
- SMALL → OBSERVE
- LARGE → SURGERY

PULMONIC STENOSIS
- MILD → OBSERVE
- LARGE → SURGERY

VSD
- SMALL → OBSERVE
- LARGE → SURGERY

COARCTATION OF AORTA
- SURGERY IF SIGNIFICANT CLINICAL HYPERTENSION

TETRALOGY OF FALLOT
- INFANCY → BLALOCK SHUNT
- LATER → DEFINITIVE SURGERY

PATENT DUCTUS
- SMALL → OBSERVE
- LARGE → PERCUTANEOUS OCCLUSION

TRANSPOSITION OF GREAT VESSELS
- INFANCY → BALLOON SEPTOSTOMY
- LATER → DEFINITIVE SURGERY

SUCCESSFUL → OBSERVE
UNSUCCESSFUL → SURGERY

CONSTIPATION

1. Barium enema, sigmoidoscopy, colonoscopy, and so on, to rule out definitive causes.
2. Remove fecal impactions.
3. Increase fluid intake to 8 glasses of clear liquids a day.
4. Increase dietary fiber.
5. Remove stimulant laxatives.
6. Bulk laxatives such as Metamucil and FiberCon.
7. Colace, Peri-Colace, and mineral oil.
8. Lactulose.
9. Subtotal colectomy for severe idiopathic constipation.

CORONARY INSUFFICIENCY

1. Confirm diagnosis by history.
2. *Acute persistent:*
   a. Hospitalize in CCU for monitoring serial EKGs and cardiac enzymes.
   b. If above studies are positive, treat as myocardial infarction (page 304).
   c. If above studies are negative, follow up with exercise tolerance test and/or thallium scan.
   d. If testing is positive, follow with coronary angiography and consider surgery. Consult cardiovascular surgeon.
   e. If testing is negative, treat risk factors [lower cholesterol (page 258), exercise, obesity, etc.]. If attacks recur, consider medical therapy with coronary vasodilators, beta blockers, or calcium channel blockers. Consider coronary angiography.
3. *Chronic recurrent:*
   a. Confirm by exercise tolerance test and thallium scan.
   b. If tests are positive and patient is physiologically young, do coronary angiography.
   c. If tests are positive and patient is old and/or a poor surgical risk, consider medical therapy with coronary vasodilators, beta blockers, or calcium channel blockers.
   d. If angiography is positive, consider angioplasty, coronary stenting, or coronary artery bypass grafting (CABG).
   e. If exercise tolerance testing or thallium scan is negative, treat medically with aspirin, vasodilators, beta blockers, and calcium channel blockers.
   f. If symptoms persist despite medical treatment, do coronary angiography anyway.
   g. If significant lesion is found, then consider coronary angioplasty, coronary stenting, or coronary bypass graft.
   h. If coronary angiography is negative, the patient may have coronary vasospasm. Treat with medical therapy and address risk factors.

Drugs and Dosage

1. *Nitrates:*
   a. Transdermal nitrates: 10–15 mg/day.
   b. Isosorbide dinitrate 5–80 mg 2–3 times per day.
   c. Nitroglycerin 0.3–0.6 mg every 15 minutes as needed.
2. *Beta blockers:*
   a. Atenolol 50–100 mg/day.
   b. Metoprolol 50–100 mg b.i.d.
3. *Calcium channel blockers:*
   a. Diltiazem 30–120 mg 3–4 times daily.
   b. Verapamil 80–120 mg 3 times daily.
   c. Nifedipine 30–80 mg 3–4 times daily.

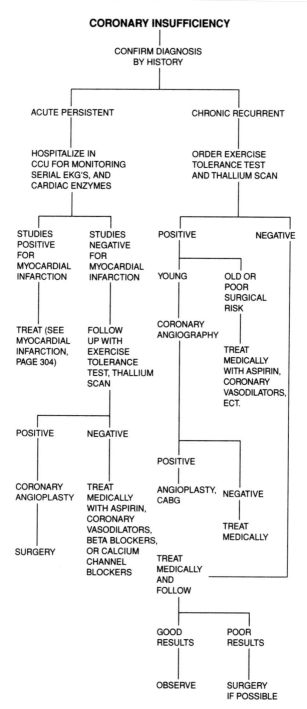

CORONARY INSUFFICIENCY

CONFIRM DIAGNOSIS
BY HISTORY

ACUTE PERSISTENT

CHRONIC RECURRENT

HOSPITALIZE IN
CCU FOR MONITORING
SERIAL EKG'S, AND
CARDIAC ENZYMES

ORDER EXERCISE
TOLERANCE TEST
AND THALLIUM SCAN

STUDIES
POSITIVE
FOR
MYOCARDIAL
INFARCTION

STUDIES
NEGATIVE
FOR
MYOCARDIAL
INFARCTION

POSITIVE

NEGATIVE

YOUNG

OLD OR
POOR
SURGICAL
RISK

TREAT (SEE
MYOCARDIAL
INFARCTION,
PAGE 304)

FOLLOW
UP WITH
EXERCISE
TOLERANCE
TEST, THALLIUM
SCAN

CORONARY
ANGIOGRAPHY

TREAT
MEDICALLY
WITH ASPIRIN,
CORONARY
VASODILATORS,
ECT.

POSITIVE

NEGATIVE

POSITIVE

CORONARY
ANGIOPLASTY

TREAT
MEDICALLY
WITH ASPIRIN,
CORONARY
VASODILATORS,
BETA BLOCKERS,
OR CALCIUM
CHANNEL
BLOCKERS

ANGIOPLASTY,
CABG

NEGATIVE

SURGERY

TREAT
MEDICALLY

TREAT
MEDICALLY
AND
FOLLOW

GOOD
RESULTS

POOR
RESULTS

OBSERVE

SURGERY
IF POSSIBLE

CREUTZFELDT–JAKOB DISEASE

1. Confirm diagnosis with EEG, CT scan or MRI, spinal fluid protein analysis, and brain biopsy. Consult a neurologist.
2. No specific therapy is available.

CRYPTOCOCCOSIS

1. Confirm diagnosis with spinal fluid analysis, India ink preparation, and culture. Consult a neurologist.
2. Treat with IV amphotericin B (0.3 mg/kg daily, initially, followed by 0.8 mg/kg every other day for 28 doses) and flucytosine 37.5 mg orally q.i.d. Treat for 6 weeks or until patient is afebrile and cultures are negative. Follow with fluconazole 200 mg/day.

CUSHING'S SYNDROME

1. Confirm diagnosis with 24-hour urine free cortisol or overnight dexamethasone suppression test.
2. *Adrenal origin:*
   a. Confirm diagnosis with plasma ACTH, high-dose dexamethasone suppression, and metyrapone test.
   b. Hyperplasia: Bilateral adrenalectomy.
   c. Adenoma—surgery.
   d. Carcinoma—surgery plus radiation and chemotherapy. Consult an oncologist.
3. *Pituitary origin:*
   a. Confirm diagnosis with plasma ACTH, metyrapone, high-dose dexamethasone suppression, CT scans, and corticotropin-releasing factor.
   b. Basophilic adenoma: Transsphenoidal resection.
   c. No tumor found at surgery: Radical hypophysectomy.
   d. Diagnosis not certain: Bilateral adrenalectomy plus irradiation of pituitary.
4. *Ectopic ACTH:*
   a. Confirm diagnosis with above studies plus x-rays and CT scans of lung and mediastinum and bronchoscopy.
   b. Bronchial adenoma: Surgery.
   c. Carcinoma of the lung: Radiation and chemotherapy. Consult an oncologist.

CUSHING'S SYNDROME

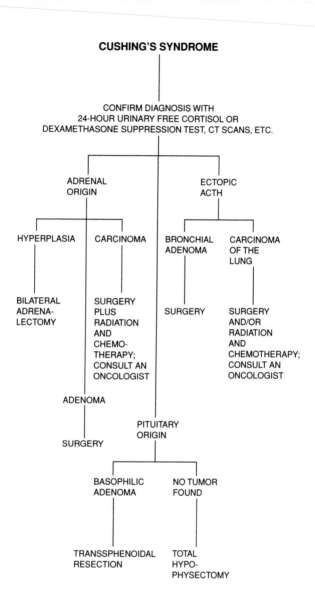

CONFIRM DIAGNOSIS WITH
24-HOUR URINARY FREE CORTISOL OR
DEXAMETHASONE SUPPRESSION TEST, CT SCANS, ETC.

ADRENAL ORIGIN

ECTOPIC ACTH

HYPERPLASIA

CARCINOMA

BRONCHIAL ADENOMA

CARCINOMA OF THE LUNG

BILATERAL ADRENA-LECTOMY

SURGERY PLUS RADIATION AND CHEMO-THERAPY; CONSULT AN ONCOLOGIST

SURGERY

SURGERY AND/OR RADIATION AND CHEMOTHERAPY; CONSULT AN ONCOLOGIST

ADENOMA

PITUITARY ORIGIN

SURGERY

BASOPHILIC ADENOMA

NO TUMOR FOUND

TRANSSPHENOIDAL RESECTION

TOTAL HYPO-PHYSECTOMY

CUTANEOUS LARVA MIGRANS

1. Confirm diagnosis with clinical picture and skin biopsy.
2. Thiabendazole 22 mg/kg b.i.d. p.o. for 5 days.
3. May also be used topically.

CYSTIC FIBROSIS

1. Confirm diagnosis with sweat test. (Chloride is typically over 70 mEq/liter.) Consult a pulmonologist.
2. Promote clearance of bronchial secretions.
3. Early antibiotics for lung infections.
4. Nutrition.
5. Observe for intestinal obstruction.

CYSTICERCOSIS

1. Confirm diagnosis with biopsy of subcutaneous nodules, skull x-rays, CT scans, and indirect hemagglutination test or CSF complement fixation test.
2. Excise cysticerci.
3. Praziquantel 20 mg/kg t.i.d. p.o. for 14 days.
4. Add 30 mg of prednisone per day to prevent drug reactions.
5. Albendazole (15 mg/kg daily for 8 days) for ocular cysticerci.
6. Surgery for ocular and CNS lesions should be considered. Consult the appropriate specialist.

CYSTINOSIS

1. Confirm diagnosis with quantitative leukocyte or cultured fibroblast cystine content.
2. Adults require no treatment.
3. Children may require treatment: Chronic renal failure (see page 412).
4. Renal transplant.

CYSTINURIA

1. Confirm diagnosis with urinary nitroprusside test.
2. Increase fluid intake to at least 4 liters/day.
3. Maintain pH of urine above 7.5 with sodium bicarbonate or acetazolamide, but watch for other types of stones.
4. Penicillamine 1–3 g/day. May reduce free cystine excretion and prevent new stone formation.

CYTOMEGALOVIRUS INFECTION

1. Confirm diagnosis by viral isolation and at least a fourfold rise in antibody titer in various serological tests.
2. Consult an oncologist or an infectious disease specialist.
3. Ganciclor quanine 5 mg/kg IV b.i.d. for 14–21 days, followed by 5 mg/kg once daily 5–7 days/week.
4. CMV immune globulin may be combined with above.
5. Foscarnet 60 mg/kg IV q.8h for 14–21 days, followed by daily IV administration of 90–120 mg/kg for maintenance.

DENGUE FEVER

1. Confirm diagnosis with hemagglutination inhibition or complement fixation tests.
2. *Treatment:* Symptomatic.
3. *Prognosis:* Mortality is negligible in the absence of hemorrhagic fever or shock.
4. *Prevention:* Mosquito control.

DEPRESSION

1. Confirm diagnosis by history and exclude medical causes of depression (endocrine disorders, dementia, etc.).
2. *Major depressive disorder:*
   a. Suicidal: Refer to psychiatrist immediately.
   b. Not suicidal: Tricyclic antidepressant, psychotherapy.
   c. Poor response: Refer to psychiatrist or try second-generation antidepressant or MAO inhibitor.
3. *Dysthymic disorder:* Tricyclic antidepressant, psychiatric consult.
4. *Bipolar disorder:*
   a. Psychiatric consult.
   b. Lithium carbonate. Monitor blood levels.
   c. If poor response to lithium, try carbamazepine or valproic acid.
5. *Involutional melancholia:* Estrogen therapy, tricyclic antidepressants, psychiatric consult.

Dosages

1. Nortriptyline 10–150 mg/day.
2. Desipramine 25–200 mg/day.
3. Fluoxetine 20–40 mg/day.
4. Paxil 20–50 mg/day.
5. Zoloft 50–200 mg/day.
6. Lithium carbonate 600–2400 mg/day.
7. Carbamazepine 800–1600 mg/day.
8. Clonazepam 1.5–6 mg/day.

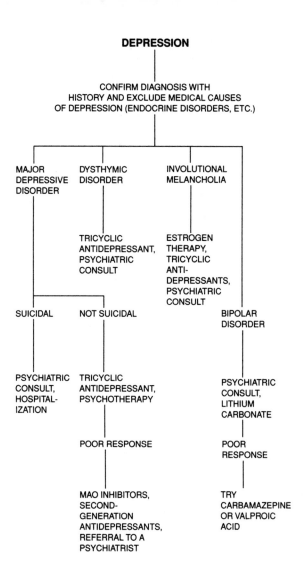

DEPRESSION

CONFIRM DIAGNOSIS WITH
HISTORY AND EXCLUDE MEDICAL CAUSES
OF DEPRESSION (ENDOCRINE DISORDERS, ETC.)

MAJOR DEPRESSIVE DISORDER

DYSTHYMIC DISORDER

TRICYCLIC ANTIDEPRESSANT, PSYCHIATRIC CONSULT

INVOLUTIONAL MELANCHOLIA

ESTROGEN THERAPY, TRICYCLIC ANTI-DEPRESSANTS, PSYCHIATRIC CONSULT

SUICIDAL

PSYCHIATRIC CONSULT, HOSPITAL-IZATION

NOT SUICIDAL

TRICYCLIC ANTIDEPRESSANT, PSYCHOTHERAPY

POOR RESPONSE

MAO INHIBITORS, SECOND-GENERATION ANTIDEPRESSANTS, REFERRAL TO A PSYCHIATRIST

BIPOLAR DISORDER

PSYCHIATRIC CONSULT, LITHIUM CARBONATE

POOR RESPONSE

TRY CARBAMAZEPINE OR VALPROIC ACID

DERMATOMYOSITIS

1. Confirm diagnosis with muscle enzymes, RA factor, ANA titer, and muscle biopsy. Look for malignancy. Consult a rheumatologist.
2. Prednisolone 40–60 mg/day, initially for 2–6 weeks, gradually tapering to low doses or alternate-day dosage.
3. Splints and physiotherapy to prevent contractures.
4. Immunosuppressants in patients who fail to respond to corticosteroids (see page 417).
5. *Prognosis:* Overall 5-year survival is estimated at 75%.

DIABETES INSIPIDUS

1. Confirm diagnosis with dehydration test (urine osmolality before and after vasopressin). Consult an endocrinologist.
2. *Pituitary diabetes insipidus:*
   a. Acute case: 5–10 units of aqueous arginine vasopressin, subcutaneously.
   b. Chronic case: Desmopressin intranasally 10–20 mcg every 12–24 hours or lypressin nasal spray every 4–6 hours.
3. *Nephrogenic diabetes insipidus:* Solute restriction, diuretics (thiazides, etc.).

DIABETES MELLITUS

1. Confirm diagnosis with FBS and glucose tolerance tests. Exclude secondary hyperglycemia (Cushing's disease, hyperthyroidism, acromegaly, etc.).
2. *Type I (insulin-dependent diabetes mellitus):*
   a. With ketoacidosis: Hospitalize and treat as outlined on page 113.
   b. Without significant ketoacidosis: Treat with diabetic diet, Humulin insulin, and glucose monitoring twice daily. If patient fails to respond, refer to an endocrinologist without delay.
3. *Type II (non-insulin-dependent diabetes mellitus):*
   a. With obesity: Treat with weight-reducing diabetic diet. Consult a dietician. If this does not control the blood sugar, add an oral hypoglycemic agent such as glipizide 2.5–10 mg/day. If that is unsuccessful, begin insulin therapy and consult an endocrinologist.
   b. Without obesity: Provide a diabetic diet. Consult a dietician. If there is no improvement, add an oral hypoglycemic agent such as glipizide 2.5–10 mg/day. If there is little or no improvement, begin insulin therapy and consult an endocrinologist.

Dosages

1. *Oral hypoglycemic agents:*
   a. Tolbutamide 500–2000 mg/day.
   b. Chlorpropamide 100–500 mg/day.
   c. Glipizide 2.5–40 mg/day.
   d. Glyburide 1.25–20 mg/day.
2. *Insulin:*
   a. Regular insulin 5–150 units/day. Peaks at 2–4 hours, lasts 5–7 hours.
   b. NPH insulin 5–150 units/day. Peaks at 6–14 hours, lasts 24 hours or more.
   c. Protamine zinc insulin 5–150 units/day. Peaks at 14–24 hours. Lasts 36 hours or more.

Tips on Giving Insulin

1. *Hyperglycemia before breakfast:* give evening dose of NPH.
2. *Late morning hyperglycemia:* Add or increase regular insulin in the morning.
3. *Late evening hyperglycemia:* Add regular insulin before dinner.
4. *Hypoglycemia at noon:* Reduce regular insulin before breakfast.
5. *Hypoglycemia in the evening:* Reduce NPH insulin before breakfast.

These are just a few examples of the many adjustments that can be made. As the clinician gains experience, he or she will develop the ingenuity to come up with many more. Remember, the number of meals, as well as the amount of calories in each meal, can be adjusted.

DIABETES MELLITUS

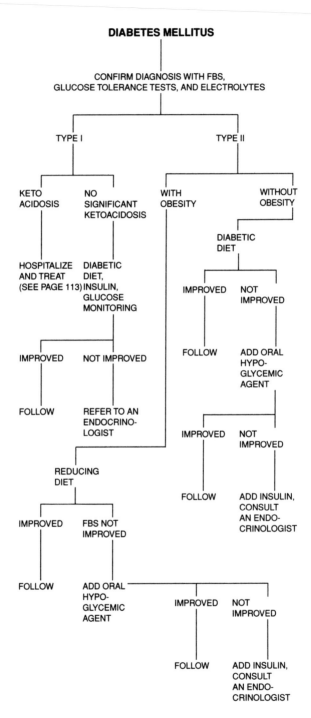

CONFIRM DIAGNOSIS WITH FBS,
GLUCOSE TOLERANCE TESTS, AND ELECTROLYTES

TYPE I

TYPE II

KETO ACIDOSIS

NO SIGNIFICANT KETOACIDOSIS

WITH OBESITY

WITHOUT OBESITY

HOSPITALIZE AND TREAT (SEE PAGE 113)

DIABETIC DIET, INSULIN, GLUCOSE MONITORING

DIABETIC DIET

IMPROVED

NOT IMPROVED

IMPROVED

NOT IMPROVED

FOLLOW

REFER TO AN ENDOCRINO-LOGIST

FOLLOW

ADD ORAL HYPO-GLYCEMIC AGENT

REDUCING DIET

IMPROVED

NOT IMPROVED

IMPROVED

FBS NOT IMPROVED

FOLLOW

ADD INSULIN, CONSULT AN ENDO-CRINOLOGIST

FOLLOW

ADD ORAL HYPO-GLYCEMIC AGENT

IMPROVED

NOT IMPROVED

FOLLOW

ADD INSULIN, CONSULT AN ENDO-CRINOLOGIST

112   Diabetes Mellitus

DIABETIC COMA

1. Confirm diagnosis by blood glucose, electrolytes, serum acetone, serum and urine osmolality, and arterial blood gases. Consult endocrinologist.
2. *Blood sugar is low:* Patient has hypoglycemic coma. Administer 50 g of 50% dextrose IV.
3. *Blood sugar is high and patient has ketoacidosis:* Patient has diabetic ketoacidosis.
   a. Dehydration: Treat with normal saline 2–5 liters initially, administered over 2–4 hours, and follow with ½ normal saline with the rate of infusion determined by urine output and serum and urine osmolality.
   b. Hyperglycemia: Treat with a bolus of 25–50 units of regular insulin initially, followed by 2–6 units/hour by infusion until ketoacidosis is resolved.
   c. Hypokalemia: This will often not be evident on the initial electrolyte report, so replacement is not usually begun until 3–4 hours after therapy has begun unless significant hypokalemia evident on first series of laboratory tests. 10–40 mEq of potassium is added to each bottle of 1000 cc of IV fluids so that the patient receives about 10 mEq of potassium per hour. Patient should not receive more than 40 mEq/hour.
   d. Acidosis: If pH is 7.1 or less or serum bicarbonate is less than 10 mEq/l., give sodium bicarbonate by adding 1 mEq/kg to the IV infusion and giving it over a 1-hour period. Repeat as needed.
4. *Ketoacidosis is absent or mild:* Patient has hyperosmolar coma.
   a. Treat initially with isotonic saline and regular insulin 2–6 units/hour. Monitor electrolytes and serum osmolality. Follow with hypotonic saline. As the blood sugar comes down, 5% glucose may be given.

DIABETIC COMA

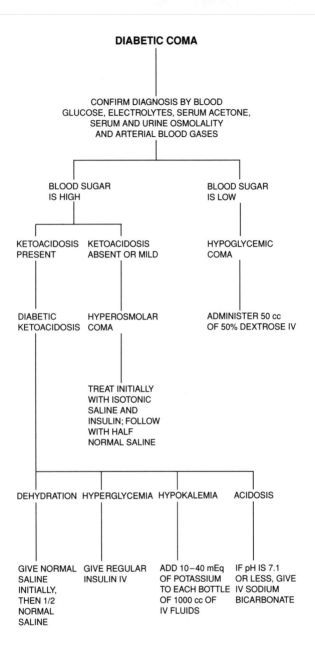

CONFIRM DIAGNOSIS BY BLOOD
GLUCOSE, ELECTROLYTES, SERUM ACETONE,
SERUM AND URINE OSMOLALITY
AND ARTERIAL BLOOD GASES

BLOOD SUGAR
IS HIGH

BLOOD SUGAR
IS LOW

KETOACIDOSIS
PRESENT

KETOACIDOSIS
ABSENT OR MILD

HYPOGLYCEMIC
COMA

DIABETIC
KETOACIDOSIS

HYPEROSMOLAR
COMA

ADMINISTER 50 cc
OF 50% DEXTROSE IV

TREAT INITIALLY
WITH ISOTONIC
SALINE AND
INSULIN; FOLLOW
WITH HALF
NORMAL SALINE

DEHYDRATION   HYPERGLYCEMIA   HYPOKALEMIA   ACIDOSIS

GIVE NORMAL
SALINE
INITIALLY,
THEN 1/2
NORMAL
SALINE

GIVE REGULAR
INSULIN IV

ADD 10–40 mEq
OF POTASSIUM
TO EACH BOTTLE
OF 1000 cc OF
IV FLUIDS

IF pH IS 7.1
OR LESS, GIVE
IV SODIUM
BICARBONATE

DIGITIALIS INTOXICATION

1. Confirm diagnosis with blood levels; get electrolytes.
2. Induce emesis if diagnosed within 1 hour of ingestion.
3. Give activated charcoal.
4. *Symptomatic bradycardia or heart block:*
   a. Give atropine 0.5 – 1.0 mg IV.
   b. Consider temporary pacemaker.
5. *Ventricular arrhythmias (consult a cardiologist):*
   a. Lidocaine 50 – 100 mg IV, followed by 1 – 4 mg/min IV drip.
   b. May use phenytoin 50 – 100 mg IV over 2 to 4 minute period, and repeat every 5 minutes as necessary up to 10 doses.
6. Use Digibind: Consult a toxicologist or a poison control center.

DIPHTHERIA

1. Confirm diagnosis by history and physical examination.
2. Administer antitoxin as soon as possible.
3. Hospitalize patients with respiratory or cutaneous diphtheria. Consider a tracheotomy.
4. Consult an infectious disease specialist.
5. Administer antibiotics to prevent spread to others.

Dosage

1. *Diphtheria antitoxin:* 20,000–100,000 units depending on stage and severity of disease. Have epinephrine available for reactions.
2. *Antibiotics:*
   a. Erythromycin 500 mg q.i.d. for 14 days.
   b. Procaine penicillin G 600,000 units q.12h. for 14 days.

Prevention

1. *Initial:* 0.5-ml DTP, four doses with the first at 6 weeks, the next two at 4- to 8-week intervals, and the last dose 6–12 months later.
2. Patients with history of diphtheria should have booster tetanus and diphtheria (Td) every 10 years for life.

DIPHYLLOBOTHRIUM LATUM

1. Confirm diagnosis with stool for ovum and parasites.
2. Praziquantel 10 mg/kg p.o. in a single dose.

DIVERTICULAR DISEASE

1. Confirm diagnosis with barium enema, sigmoidoscopy, or colonoscopy.
2. *Uncomplicated diverticulosis:* Treat with high-fiber diet, psyllium supplement. Follow for complications.
3. *Complications:*
   a. Diverticulitis:
      - Confirm diagnosis with CT scans, ultrasound, and flat plate and upright of abdomen to rule out perforations. Consult a gastroenterologist. May need gallium scan to exclude abscess.
      - Bowel rest, IV fluids, IV antibiotics (cefuroxime 1 g q.12h. plus metronidazole 500 mg t.i.d.); or perhaps use oral antibiotics (ciprofloxacin 500 mg b.i.d. plus metronidazole).
      - Symptoms persist: Consult a surgeon.
      - Symptoms improve: Follow up with treatment for diverticulosis.
      - Recurrent attacks: Bowel resection.
   b. Bleeding diverticula:
      - Bowel rest, IV fluids, transfusions, consult a gastroenterologist.
      - Symptoms persist: Consult a gastroenterologist for selective arterial vasopressin, or consult a surgeon for resection.
      - Improves: Follow up with treatment for diverticulosis. Correct anemia.
   c. Fistula: Consult a surgeon.

DIVERTICULAR DISEASE

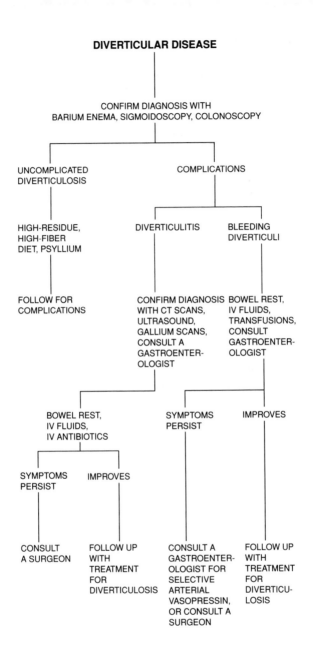

CONFIRM DIAGNOSIS WITH
BARIUM ENEMA, SIGMOIDOSCOPY, COLONOSCOPY

UNCOMPLICATED
DIVERTICULOSIS

COMPLICATIONS

HIGH-RESIDUE,
HIGH-FIBER
DIET, PSYLLIUM

DIVERTICULITIS

BLEEDING
DIVERTICULI

FOLLOW FOR
COMPLICATIONS

CONFIRM DIAGNOSIS
WITH CT SCANS,
ULTRASOUND,
GALLIUM SCANS,
CONSULT A
GASTROENTER-
OLOGIST

BOWEL REST,
IV FLUIDS,
TRANSFUSIONS,
CONSULT
GASTROENTER-
OLOGIST

BOWEL REST,
IV FLUIDS,
IV ANTIBIOTICS

SYMPTOMS
PERSIST

IMPROVES

SYMPTOMS
PERSIST

IMPROVES

CONSULT
A SURGEON

FOLLOW UP
WITH
TREATMENT
FOR
DIVERTICULOSIS

CONSULT A
GASTROENTER-
OLOGIST FOR
SELECTIVE
ARTERIAL
VASOPRESSIN,
OR CONSULT A
SURGEON

FOLLOW UP
WITH
TREATMENT
FOR
DIVERTICU-
LOSIS

DOWN'S SYNDROME

1. Confirm diagnosis by history and physical examination and chromosomal analysis.
2. Treatment is supportive because there is no specific treatment. Treat complications such as cataracts and cardiac anomalies by appropriate surgery.

DRACUNCULIASIS

1. Confirm diagnosis with eosinophilia, elevated serum IgE, and antifilarial antibody.
2. Metronidazole 500 mg t.i.d. for 5 days, or diethylcarbamazine 6 mg/kg daily for 2 weeks.
3. Retreatment required in up to one-quarter of patients.

DRESSLER'S SYNDROME

1. Confirm diagnosis with CBC, sedimentation rate, EKG, and friction rub. Consult a cardiologist.
2. Aspirin or other NSAIDs.
3. If NSAIDs fail, use systemic corticosteroids such as prednisone 60 mg daily for 3 weeks and taper over 6-week period. Avoid anticoagulants.

DRUG INTOXICATION

1. Confirm diagnosis by history, blood or urine tests for the drug, CBC, chemistry panels, and response to the antidote.
2. Support vital signs with oxygen, airway, appropriate intravenous fluids, CPR. Consult a toxicologist or an acute care specialist.
3. Withdraw the drug and, where appropriate, gastrointestinal decontamination with syrup of ipecac, gastric lavage, activated charcoal, or catharsis.
4. Assist in rapid elimination of the drug with forced diuresis (oral or IV), chelation therapy, or alteration of urinary pH. Consider peritoneal dialysis or renal dialysis.
5. Administer appropriate antidote. Call a poison control center for guidance.

DRUG REACTIONS

1. Confirm diagnosis by history, skin testing, and RAST.
2. Withdraw or avoid the drug.
3. Treat anaphylactic reactions with epinephrine, antihistamines, steroids, IV fluids, and CPR (page 59).
4. Treat serum sickness with antihistamines and steroids (page 441).
5. Treat skin reactions with local and systemic steroids (page 129, Eczema, etc.).

DUBIN–JOHNSON SYNDROME

1. Confirm diagnosis with liver function tests, urine porphyrins, and liver biopsy.
2. Avoid oral contraceptives.
3. No specific treatment is available.

EATON–LAMBERT SYNDROME

1. Confirm diagnosis with electromyography and tests for carcinoma of the lung.
2. Treat the neoplasm (page 56).
3. Consult neurologist.
4. *Anticholinesterase drugs:* Pyridostigmine 60 mg t.i.d. and gradually increase the dose using endrophonium testing to evaluate need for dosage increase.
5. Guanidine 20–30 mg/kg daily in three to four divided doses. Follow with CBC, chemistry panel, and pancreatic function tests weekly.
6. 4-Aminopyridine 40–200 mg/day. Watch for side effects of cardiovascular, gastrointestinal, and nervous systems.
7. Corticosteroids (such as prednisone 60 mg/day) for 3 weeks and gradually taper.
8. Immunosuppressants such as azathioprine 1.5–2.5 mg/kg daily for at least 2 months before giving up.
9. *Plasmapheresis:* Consult a neurologist.

ECHINOCOCCOSIS

1. Confirm diagnosis with chest x-rays, CT scans, ultrasound, and serological tests.
2. *Symptomatic cysts:* Consult a surgeon for resection. Pretreatment with albendazole may be advisable.
3. *Asymptomatic cysts:* Albendazole 400 mg b.i.d. for 28 days and repeat. Follow treatment with surgery in persistent cases. Consult an infectious disease specialist.

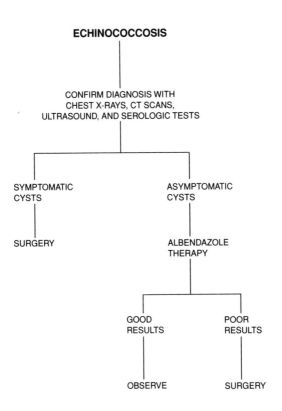

ECTOPIC PREGNANCY

1. Confirm diagnosis with serum B–hCG immunoassay, pelvic ultrasound, and culdocentesis. A peritoneal tap may be useful.
2. Consult a gynecologist for surgery.

ECZEMA

1. Confirm diagnosis with family history, skin testing, skin biopsy and dermatology consult.
2. First try eliminating allergens from the diet or environment. Lubricate skin with non-perfumed bath oil, petrolatum or Eucerin. Eliminate environmental stress. Consult psychiatrist.
3. If above measures unsuccessful, treat with antihistamines such as hydroxyzine 25–50 mg q.i.d. or diphenhydramine 25–50 mg q.i.d.
4. If above measures unsuccessful, treat with topical corticosteroids such as hydrocortisone acetate 1% cream, triamcinolone acetonide 0.1% cream or 0.05% fluocinonide cream. Do not use the stronger corticosteroid cream on the face.
5. If above treatment is ineffective, consult a dermatologist or allergist for desensitization to specific allergens.

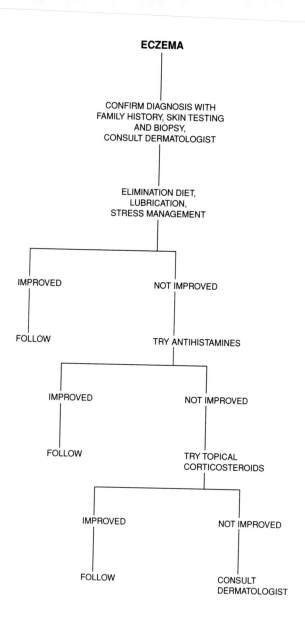

ECZEMA

CONFIRM DIAGNOSIS WITH
FAMILY HISTORY, SKIN TESTING
AND BIOPSY,
CONSULT DERMATOLOGIST

ELIMINATION DIET,
LUBRICATION,
STRESS MANAGEMENT

IMPROVED

NOT IMPROVED

FOLLOW

TRY ANTIHISTAMINES

IMPROVED

NOT IMPROVED

FOLLOW

TRY TOPICAL
CORTICOSTEROIDS

IMPROVED

NOT IMPROVED

FOLLOW

CONSULT
DERMATOLOGIST

EHLERS–DANLOS SYNDROME

1. Confirm diagnosis with clinical evaluation and consultation with a rheumatologist.
2. No specific therapy available. Consult a rheumatologist, an orthopedic surgeon, and a dermatologist for specific problems.

EMPHYSEMA

1. Confirm diagnosis with chest x-ray, spirometry, and arterial blood gases.
2. *Acute:*
   a. Consult pulmonologist.
   b. Hospitalization.
   c. Low-flow oxygen therapy, IPPB with inhaled bronchodilators (terbutaline 500 µg q.2h., albuterol or metaproterenol q.1–2h.), and IV aminophylline (0.5 mg/kg per hour). Consult a respiratory therapist.
   d. If no improvement, add antibiotics and oral corticosteroids (prednisone 60 mg/day and taper) or IV corticosteroids (Decadron 4–8 mg IV q.6h).
   e. If no improvement, consider endotracheal intubation.
3. *Chronic:*
   a. Stop smoking.
   b. Inhaled bronchodilators (ipratropium bromide 18–72 µg q.6h or terbutaline 500 µg q.4h).
   c. Oral bronchodilators (albuterol syrup or tablets 2–4 mg q.i.d. or theophylline extended-release capsules or tablets 200–600 mg/day).
   d. If there is no improvement, consult a pulmonologist for use of oral corticosteroids, home oxygen, and physiotherapy.
   e. If there is no improvement, consider a lung transplant.

EMPHYSEMA

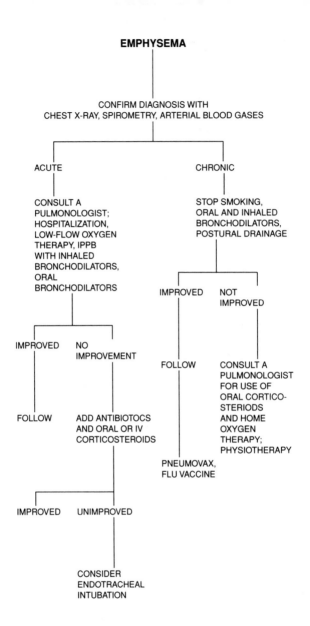

CONFIRM DIAGNOSIS WITH
CHEST X-RAY, SPIROMETRY, ARTERIAL BLOOD GASES

ACUTE

CONSULT A
PULMONOLOGIST;
HOSPITALIZATION,
LOW-FLOW OXYGEN
THERAPY, IPPB
WITH INHALED
BRONCHODILATORS,
ORAL
BRONCHODILATORS

IMPROVED   NO
IMPROVEMENT

FOLLOW   ADD ANTIBIOTOCS
AND ORAL OR IV
CORTICOSTEROIDS

IMPROVED   UNIMPROVED

CONSIDER
ENDOTRACHEAL
INTUBATION

CHRONIC

STOP SMOKING,
ORAL AND INHALED
BRONCHODILATORS,
POSTURAL DRAINAGE

IMPROVED   NOT
IMPROVED

FOLLOW   CONSULT A
PULMONOLOGIST
FOR USE OF
ORAL CORTICO-
STERIODS
AND HOME
OXYGEN
THERAPY;
PHYSIOTHERAPY

PNEUMOVAX,
FLU VACCINE

Emphysema   133

EMPYEMA OF THE LUNG

1. Confirm diagnosis by routine chest x-ray with lateral decubitus and thoracentesis with smear and culture.
2. Antibiotics appropriate to the smear and culture (see page 370).
3. Consult a thoracic surgeon for tube thoracostomy.
4. If drainage is inadequate, consider loculation of fluid and administer streptokinase 250,000 units or urokinase 100,000 units intrapleurally.
5. If symptoms and signs persist, consider open thoracotomy.

ENCEPHALITIS, VIRAL

1. Confirm diagnosis by CSF examination; look for herpes simplex virus DNA in the CSF by PCR. Do CT scans and MRIs when indicated. Consult a neurologist.
2. *Herpes simplex encephalitis:* Acyclovir IV 10 mg/kg q.8h. for 10 days.
3. *Arbor virus encephalitis:* No specific treatment available. Supportive care as indicated.

ENCEPHALOMYELITIS, ACUTE DISSEMINATED

1. Confirm diagnosis by history of recent vaccination or exanthematous illness, spinal fluid analysis, and MRI examination. Consult a neurologist.
2. Methylprednisolone 1000 mg IV daily (administered over 4- to 6-hour period) for 3 days followed by oral prednisolone 1 mg/kg daily for 14 days. Consult a neurologist for other protocols.
3. ACTH may be tried. Consult a neurologist for protocol.

EOSINOPHILIC PNEUMONIA

1. Confirm diagnosis by chest x-ray, sputum analysis, CBC, and tests to rule out parasites.
2. Treatment of parasites and other causative organisms.
3. Corticosteroids may be tried for the idiopathic type. Prednisone 1 mg/kg daily is a suitable therapeutic agent. This may be gradually tapered once clinical remission is achieved.

EPIDIDYMITIS

1. Confirm diagnosis with clinical observation and urethral smear and culture.
2. *Gonococcal epididymitis:* Ceftriaxone 250 mg IM, followed by doxycycline 100 mg b.i.d. p.o. for 10 days.
3. *Chlamydial epididymitis:* Doxycycline 100 mg b.i.d. for 10 days.
4. *Nonspecific epididymitis:* Treat as gonococcal form.
5. Rapid identification of sexual partners to prevent the spread of this disease.

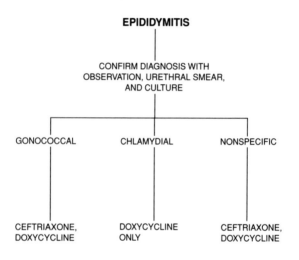

EPIDURAL ABSCESS

1. Confirm diagnosis by MRI or CT scan. Look for diabetes mellitus and other systemic disease.
2. Start IV cephalosporin such as cefuroxime 0.75–1.5 grams q.8h.
3. Consult a neurosurgeon for immediate decompression and drainage.
4. Determine ultimate antibiotic therapy based on culture and sensitivity.

EPILEPSY, IDIOPATHIC

1. Confirm diagnosis by history, EEG, CT scans, or MRIs.
2. *Grand mal, focal cortical, or complex partial seizures:*
   a. Try monotherapy with either phenytoin, carbamazepine, valproic acid, or phenobarbital.
   b. If poor control, push single drug to maximum dose while monitoring blood levels and side effects.
   c. If poor control continues, try combinations of first-line drugs. For example, phenytoin and carbamazepine or phenytoin and phenobarbital.
   d. If poor control continues, add to or replace first-line drug with second-line drug (clonazepam, primidone, gabapentin, lamotrigine).
   e. If poor control persists, refer to special center for surgery of cortical focus.
3. *Petit mal:*
   a. If patient has only absence seizures, try ethosuximide first.
   b. If patient has mixed seizure disorder, try valproic acid first.
   c. If there is a poor response from the above drugs, patient should be given a trial of clonazepam or phenobarbital.
   d. If there is a poor response to above drugs, then try trimethadione or consult a neurologist to reevaluate the diagnosis.
4. *Cessation of therapy:* If patient is seizure-free for 5 or more years, slow withdrawal of medication may be tried. Consult a neurologist.

Dosages

1. *Phenytoin:* 100–600 mg/day in single or divided doses. Available in chewables, liquid, or capsules.
2. *Carbamazepine:* 200–1200 mg/day in divided doses b.i.d. to q.i.d. Available in chewable form, as well as scored tablets.
3. *Phenobarbital:* 30–120 mg/day in single or di-

vided dose. Available in liquid and tablet form.
4. *Valproate:* 250–1250 mg/day in divided doses. Available in capsules, tablets, and sprinkle form.
5. *Clonazepam:* 0.25–5.0 mg/day in divided doses. Available in tablets.
6. *Ethosuximide:* 250–1250 mg/day, in divided doses b.i.d. Available in capsules.
7. *Primidone:* 500–1000 mg/day. Available in tablets.
8. *Trimethadione:* 900–2100 mg/day in divided doses. Available in tablets.
9. *Lamotrigine:* 300–500 mg/day. Available in tablets or capsules. Begin therapy with low dose to avoid side effects.
10. *Gabapentin:* 900–1200 mg/day in divided doses. Available in capsules.

EPILEPSY, IDIOPATHIC

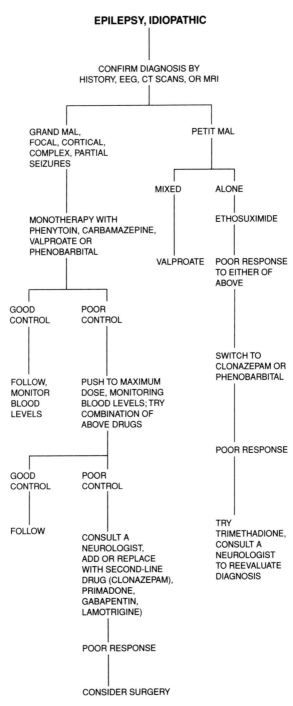

CONFIRM DIAGNOSIS BY
HISTORY, EEG, CT SCANS, OR MRI

GRAND MAL,
FOCAL, CORTICAL,
COMPLEX, PARTIAL
SEIZURES

PETIT MAL

MIXED   ALONE

MONOTHERAPY WITH
PHENYTOIN, CARBAMAZEPINE,
VALPROATE OR
PHENOBARBITAL

ETHOSUXIMIDE

VALPROATE   POOR RESPONSE
TO EITHER OF
ABOVE

GOOD   POOR
CONTROL   CONTROL

FOLLOW,   PUSH TO MAXIMUM
MONITOR   DOSE, MONITORING
BLOOD   BLOOD LEVELS; TRY
LEVELS   COMBINATION OF
              ABOVE DRUGS

SWITCH TO
CLONAZEPAM OR
PHENOBARBITAL

GOOD   POOR
CONTROL   CONTROL

POOR RESPONSE

FOLLOW

CONSULT A
NEUROLOGIST,
ADD OR REPLACE
WITH SECOND-LINE
DRUG (CLONAZEPAM),
PRIMADONE,
GABAPENTIN,
LAMOTRIGINE)

TRY
TRIMETHADIONE,
CONSULT A
NEUROLOGIST
TO REEVALUATE
DIAGNOSIS

POOR RESPONSE

CONSIDER SURGERY

EPILEPSY, STATUS

1. Confirm diagnosis with history and clinical observation. Consult a neurologist.
2. Establish airway, set up an IV line, and do CBC, chemistry and electrolyte panel, and arterial blood gases.
3. Lorazepam IV, 0.1 mg/kg at the rate of 2 mg/min, or diazepam 0.15 mg/kg at the rate of 3–5 mg/min. Watch for respiratory depression.
4. Simultaneously start phenytoin in a loading dose of 20 mg/kg, given at 50 mg/min. A new compound, fosphenytoin can be given even faster.
5. If seizures persist, consult an anesthesiologist for endotracheal intubation and give phenobarbital 15 mg/kg at 100 mg/min.
6. If seizures persist, consult a neurologist for paraldehyde and consult an anesthesiologist for general anesthetic.
7. Transfer to ICU.

ERYSIPELAS

1. Confirm diagnosis with clinical evaluation, blood culture, or culture of exudate. Surgical exploration may be needed.
2. Aqueous penicillin 1–2 million units IV q.4h. or erythromycin 500 mg q.6h. p.o. or vancomycin 1 g IV q.12hs. Another alternative is cefoxitin 1–2 g IV q.8h.

ERYTHEMA MULTIFORME

1. Confirm diagnosis by clinical examination, dermatology consult, and biopsy.
2. Withdraw offending agent (drugs, etc.).
3. Supportive measures for mild cases.
4. If Stevens–Johnson syndrome develops, nasogastric or intravenous feeding may be necessary.
5. Consult a dermatologist before using corticosteroids or immunosuppressants.
6. If there is eye involvement, consult an ophthalmologist without delay.

ERYTHEMA NODOSUM

1. Confirm diagnosis by clinical evaluation, dermatology consult, and biopsy.
2. Eliminate offending agent (drugs, etc.).
3. Bedrest.
4. Oral NSAIDs.
5. Systemic corticosteroids for persistent cases, such as prednisone 60 mg/day and gradually tapering over 4- to 6-week period. Consult a dermatologist before starting this aggressive therapy.

ESOPHAGEAL CARCINOMA

1. Confirm diagnosis with barium swallow, esophagoscopy, and biopsy. Evaluate extent of spread by CT scans and ultrasonography.
2. *Squamous cell carcinoma:* Surgical resection, followed by chemotherapy. Consult an oncologist.
3. *Adenocarcinoma:* Resection rarely produces cure.
4. Palliative measures may be advisable and include mechanical dilatation, radiotherapy, gastrostomy, or prosthetic bypass of tumor.
5. *Prognosis:* Five-year survival after surgery is less than 5%.

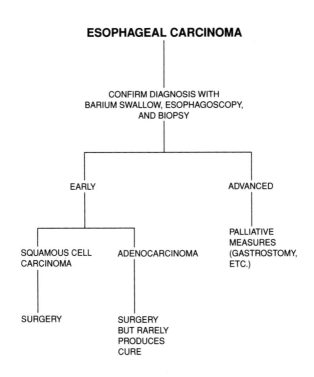

ESOPHAGEAL CARCINOMA

CONFIRM DIAGNOSIS WITH
BARIUM SWALLOW, ESOPHAGOSCOPY,
AND BIOPSY

EARLY

ADVANCED

PALLIATIVE
MEASURES
(GASTROSTOMY,
ETC.)

SQUAMOUS CELL
CARCINOMA

ADENOCARCINOMA

SURGERY

SURGERY
BUT RARELY
PRODUCES
CURE

ESOPHAGEAL VARICES

1. Confirm diagnosis by esophagoscopy, liver function tests, and celiac and mesenteric arteriography. Consult a gastroenterologist.
2. Type and cross-match 6 units of blood and administer appropriate amounts to keep blood pressure at 90-mm systolic or better. May give collodial solutions or normal saline until blood is ready.
3. Vasopressin intravenously, 0.4 units per minute until bleeding stops or for 24 hours and then 0.2 units per minute for an additional 24 hours. Because vasopressin induces generalized vasoconstriction, including coronary vasoconstriction, transdermal nitroglycerin is given concurrently.
4. If vasopressin is not successful, octreotide (which is synthetic somatostatin) is given 50 μg stat IV and 50 μg hourly.
5. If above ineffective, then consult a gastroenterologist for sclerotherapy.
6. If bleeding is marked and sclerotherapy is not feasible, pass Sengstaken–Blakemore tube. Use gastric balloon only at first, and then use esophageal balloon if gastric balloon alone is ineffective. Deflate esophageal balloon for 10 minutes every 3 hours to prevent mucosal damage.
7. As an alternative to the Sengstaken–Blakemore tube, transjugular intrahepatic portal–systemic stent shunt (TIPSS) may be done. A stent is placed between the portal and hepatic vein under radiologic control. Consult a radiologist.
8. Consult a surgeon for esophageal transection with a stapling gun.
9. Prevention of recurrent bleeding may be done by sclerotherapy, bonding, TIPSS, or portacaval shunt surgery.

ESOPHAGEAL VARICES

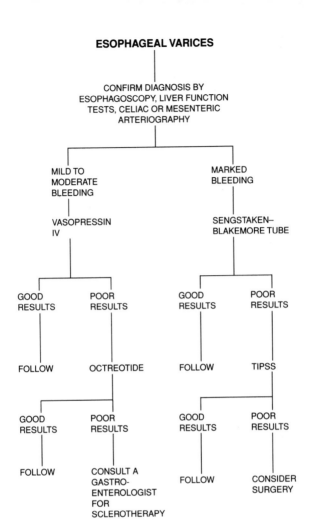

CONFIRM DIAGNOSIS BY
ESOPHAGOSCOPY, LIVER FUNCTION
TESTS, CELIAC OR MESENTERIC
ARTERIOGRAPHY

MILD TO MODERATE BLEEDING

VASOPRESSIN IV

GOOD RESULTS → FOLLOW

POOR RESULTS → OCTREOTIDE

GOOD RESULTS → FOLLOW

POOR RESULTS → CONSULT A GASTRO-ENTEROLOGIST FOR SCLEROTHERAPY

MARKED BLEEDING

SENGSTAKEN–BLAKEMORE TUBE

GOOD RESULTS → FOLLOW

POOR RESULTS → TIPSS

GOOD RESULTS → FOLLOW

POOR RESULTS → CONSIDER SURGERY

Esophageal Varices   149

ESSENTIAL HYPERTENSION

1. Confirm diagnosis by history and excluding secondary causes of hypertension.
2. *Acute hypertensive crisis:*
   a. Moderate: Treat with nifedipine (10–20 mg, chewable) or IV labetalol (2 mg/min to a maximum of 200 mg).
   b. Severe: Hospitalize and get cardiology consult to assist in IV nitroprusside administration.
   c. Complicated by cerebral hemorrhage, heart failure, or renal failure; see pages 187, 241, and 410 and consult appropriate specialist.
3. *Chronic hypertension:*
   a. Mild: Treat with salt restriction, weight loss, exercise, and avoidance of smoking and alcohol. If symptoms persist, add diuretic, hydrochlorothiazide 50 mg/day. Cover potassium loss with potassium supplement or diet. If diuretic is ineffective, treat as moderate to severe.
   b. Moderate to severe: Start with a beta blocker such as atenolol 50–100 mg/day or a calcium channel blocker such as verapamil 60–80 mg t.i.d. This is also available in a long-acting form. If the above drugs are ineffective, a diuretic (hydrochlorothiazide 50 mg/day or ACE inhibitor (lisinopril 10–20 mg/day) may be added.
4. *Resistant chronic hypertension:* A vasodilator drug such as hydralazine 25–75 mg t.i.d. or minoxidil 10–50 mg/day may be added. It is wise to consult a cardiologist, endocrinologist, or a nephrologist to look for secondary hypertension.

ESSENTIAL HYPERTENSION

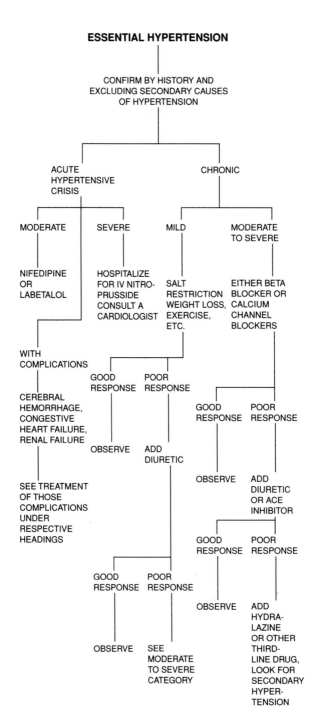

CONFIRM BY HISTORY AND
EXCLUDING SECONDARY CAUSES
OF HYPERTENSION

ACUTE HYPERTENSIVE CRISIS

CHRONIC

MODERATE

NIFEDIPINE OR LABETALOL

SEVERE

HOSPITALIZE FOR IV NITRO-PRUSSIDE CONSULT A CARDIOLOGIST

MILD

SALT RESTRICTION WEIGHT LOSS, EXERCISE, ETC.

MODERATE TO SEVERE

EITHER BETA BLOCKER OR CALCIUM CHANNEL BLOCKERS

WITH COMPLICATIONS

CEREBRAL HEMORRHAGE, CONGESTIVE HEART FAILURE, RENAL FAILURE

SEE TREATMENT OF THOSE COMPLICATIONS UNDER RESPECTIVE HEADINGS

GOOD RESPONSE

POOR RESPONSE

OBSERVE

ADD DIURETIC

GOOD RESPONSE

POOR RESPONSE

OBSERVE

ADD DIURETIC OR ACE INHIBITOR

GOOD RESPONSE

POOR RESPONSE

OBSERVE

ADD HYDRA-LAZINE OR OTHER THIRD-LINE DRUG, LOOK FOR SECONDARY HYPER-TENSION

GOOD RESPONSE

POOR RESPONSE

OBSERVE

SEE MODERATE TO SEVERE CATEGORY

Essential Hypertension   151

EXTRADURAL HEMATOMA

1. Confirm diagnosis with CT scans or MRIs.
2. Consult a neurosurgeon for surgical evacuation of the clot.
3. Consider prophylactic anticonvulsants following surgery.

FABRY'S DISEASE

1. Confirm diagnosis by clinical evaluation and skin or renal biopsy. Consult an ophthalmologist or a dermatologist.
2. Warn patient regarding the risks of hypohidrosis.
3. Treat painful neuropathy with phenytoin 200−600 mg/day.
4. Treat renal failure with chronic dialysis or renal transplant.
5. Consider enzyme replacement therapy.

FAMILIAL MEDITERRANEAN FEVER

1. Confirm diagnosis by family history and ethnic background.
2. No specific treatment is effective during an attack.
3. Colchicine 0.6 mg b.i.d. to t.i.d. p.o. will reduce the frequency of attacks.

FAMILIAL PERIODIC PARALYSIS

1. Confirm diagnosis by family history, electrolyte determination during attacks, and response to treatment.
2. *Hypokalemic form:* Treat with rapid ingestion of 20–100 mEq of KCL in a suitable form during attack.
3. *Hyperkalemic form:* Administer calcium gluconate, glucose, and insulin during attack.
4. Reduce the number of attacks with acetazolamide 250–1000 mg/day.

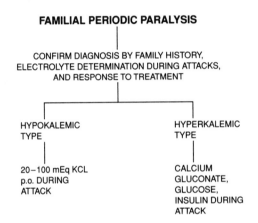

FAMILIAL PERIODIC PARALYSIS

CONFIRM DIAGNOSIS BY FAMILY HISTORY, ELECTROLYTE DETERMINATION DURING ATTACKS, AND RESPONSE TO TREATMENT

HYPOKALEMIC TYPE

20–100 mEq KCL p.o. DURING ATTACK

HYPERKALEMIC TYPE

CALCIUM GLUCONATE, GLUCOSE, INSULIN DURING ATTACK

FANCONI SYNDROME

1. Confirm diagnosis by urinalysis for amino acids and glucose. Look for cause (Wilson's disease, cystinosis, etc.). Renal biopsy may be necessary. Consult a nephrologist.
2. Liberal water, sodium, and potassium intake to replace deficits.
3. Alkali (sodium bicarbonate 0.5–2.0 mmol/kg daily) supplements to correct metabolic acidosis.
4. Vitamin D should be given to restore bone.

FIBROMYALGIA

1. Confirm diagnosis by history and physical examination and exclusion of other disorders. Consult a rheumatologist.
2. Exercise program such as jogging or fast walking, beginning at 1 mile three times a week and increasing to 3–5 miles three times a week.
3. Antidepressants such as imipramine 25–100 mg h.s. or amitriptyline 10–150 mg h.s.
4. Trigger point injections with 2–4 cc of 1–2% lidocaine and 0.5 cc of triamcinolone (40 mg/cc). No more frequently than monthly to avoid Cushing's syndrome. Lidocaine injections alone may be successful.
5. Psychotherapy.

FILARIASIS

1. Confirm diagnosis by blood, lymph, urine, or tissue smear and slit-lamp examination. Serology may be necessary.
2. *Wuchereria bancrofti:* Single dose of ivermectin 20 µg/kg p.o.
3. *Onchocerciasis:* Single dose of ivermectin 150 µg/kg p.o.
4. *Loa loa:* Diethylcarbamazine 9–12 mg/kg daily in three divided doses for 14–21 days. Begin with 50 mg/day and gradually increase to the full dose, watching for allergic reactions. Be ready to give antihistamines and corticosteroids for allergic phenomena.
5. Repeat doses to be sure the adult worm is eradicated. This is every 6–12 months for *W. bancrofti* and onchocerciasis and at 4- to 6-week intervals for Loa loa.
6. Lymphedema may be treated with compression garments, surgery, or coumarin 400 mg q.24h.

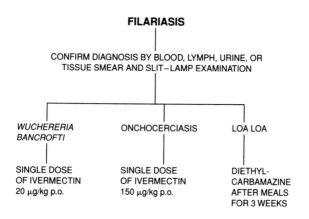

FRACTURES

1. Confirm diagnosis by x-rays, CT scans, or bone scans.
2. Apply cold packs (if under 24 hours old) or hot packs (if over 24 hours old) and immobilize with a splint or similar device.
3. In fractures of the skull and spine, consult a neurosurgeon.
4. In all other fractures, consult an orthopedic surgeon.

FUNGAL INFECTIONS OF THE SKIN

1. Confirm diagnosis with KOH preparations, cultures and Wood's lamp. Consult a dermatologist for persistent cases.
2. *Dermatophyte infections:*
   a. Tinea capitis: Griseofulvin 10–15 mg/kg p.o. daily after meals for 6–8 weeks.
   b. Tinea corporis: Topical imidazole cream daily. Continue for 2 weeks after disappearance of lesions.
   c. Tinea pedis: Topical imidazole cream daily. Continue for 3 months. Alternatively, try undecylenic acid ointment twice daily for 3 months. Stubborn cases may require griseofulvin 500 mg b.i.d. or ketoconazole 200–400 mg daily. Tinea manum requires oral therapy also.
   d. Onychomycosis: Griseofulvin 500 mg b.i.d. for 4–6 months for fingernails and 12–24 months for toenails. Alternatively, ketoconazole 200–400 mg/day may be used. Terbinafine HCL 250 mg a day may be successful in 3–6 months.
3. *Candida:* Topical amphotericin B cream, lotion, or ointment once or twice daily works well. Alternatively, nystatin, imidazoles, and ciclopirox may be used. Oral nystatin may be necessary to prevent reseeding of involved areas.
4. *Tinea versicolor:* Selenium sulfide suspension twice weekly and allowed to dry and remain on overnight. It is showered off in the morning. For persistent cases, ketoconazole is given 400 mg once a week 2 hours before exercise.

Preparations

1. *Imidazole:* Lotrimin, Mycelex cream, lotion, Gyne-Lotrimin cream.
2. *Griseofulvin:* Fulvicin U/F, P/G tablets.
3. *Amphotericin B:* Fungizone cream, lotion, ointment.
4. *Ciclopirox:* Loprox cream.
5. *Ketoconazole:* Oral tablets.
6. *Nystatin:* Mycostatin cream, lotion, intravaginal tablets.

FUNGAL INFECTIONS OF THE SKIN

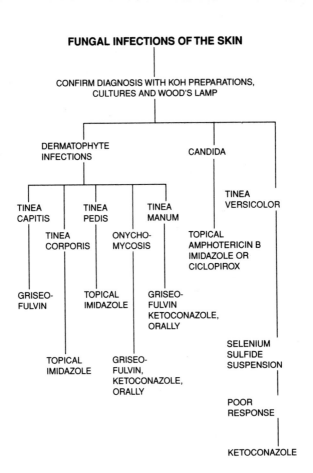

CONFIRM DIAGNOSIS WITH KOH PREPARATIONS,
CULTURES AND WOOD'S LAMP

DERMATOPHYTE
INFECTIONS

CANDIDA

TINEA
VERSICOLOR

TINEA
CAPITIS

TINEA
PEDIS

TINEA
MANUM

TINEA
CORPORIS

ONYCHO-
MYCOSIS

TOPICAL
AMPHOTERICIN B
IMIDAZOLE OR
CICLOPIROX

GRISEO-
FULVIN

TOPICAL
IMIDAZOLE

GRISEO-
FULVIN
KETOCONAZOLE,
ORALLY

SELENIUM
SULFIDE
SUSPENSION

TOPICAL
IMIDAZOLE

GRISEO-
FULVIN,
KETOCONAZOLE,
ORALLY

POOR
RESPONSE

KETOCONAZOLE

GALACTOSEMIA

1. Confirm diagnosis by red cell analysis of galactose-1-phosphate uridylyltransferase (GALT) and elevated blood and urine galactose.
2. Treat with galactose-free diet, especially avoiding milk. Milk substitutes may be used.

GAS GANGRENE

1. Confirm diagnosis by clinical evaluation, smear and culture of exudates, x-rays of soft tissue, or frozen section biopsy.
2. Treat with intravenous aqueous penicillin G 20 million units daily. Calculate lower doses for children. Alternatives are chloramphenicol 4 g/day or a cephalosporin.
3. Localized infections of the skin may be treated by débridement.

GASTRITIS

1. Confirm diagnosis by gastroscopy and biopsy with urease testing.
2. Treat hemorrhage with infusion of saline solution containing 12 mg of norepinephrine bitartrate per 200 ml. Transfusions for large hemorrhages.
3. Treat erosive gastritis with oral antacid therapy hourly or IV H2 antagonists such as ranitidine 150–300 mg q.12h. IV.
4. Treat *H. pylori* gastritis with amoxicillin 500 mg q.i.d., metronidazole 500 mg t.i.d. and bismuth subsalicylate 2 tablets q.i.d. for 2–3 weeks.
5. No treatment is necessary for chronic gastritis unless there is associated pernicious anemia (see page 351).

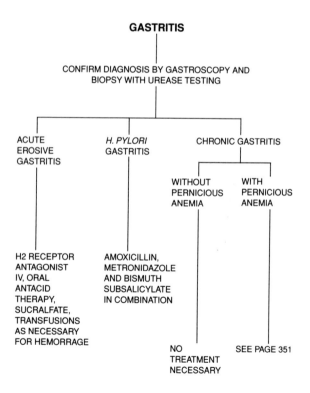

GASTROENTERITIS

1. Confirm diagnosis with stool smear for leukocytes, cultures, and ovum and parasites.
2. If patient is severely ill with more than six stools/hour and vomiting, hospitalize for IV fluids, antiemetics (such as prochlorperazine 12.5–25 mg q.6h. IM), and diphenoxylate HCl.
3. If not severely ill and less than six stools per hour with minimal vomiting, patient may be treated at home with a balanced electrolyte solution such as two level teaspoons of salt and 50 g of glucose to each quart of water or 5% glucose and half normal saline solution.
4. Once organism is isolated, antibiotics may be administered:

    For *Salmonella:* Ciprofloxacin 200 mg q.12h. IV.

    For *Shigella:* Ciprofloxacin 500 mg q.12h. p.o.

    For traveler's diarrhea: Doxycycline 100 mg q.12h. p.o.

    For *Campylobacter:* Erythromycin 500 mg q.6h. p.o.

    For Giardia: Mitronidazole 250 mg t.i.d. p.o.
5. Antibiotics are unnecessary if patient has recovered.

GASTROENTERITIS

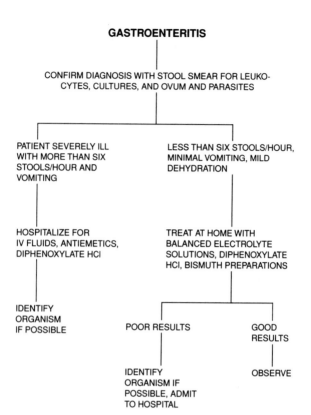

CONFIRM DIAGNOSIS WITH STOOL SMEAR FOR LEUKO-
CYTES, CULTURES, AND OVUM AND PARASITES

PATIENT SEVERELY ILL
WITH MORE THAN SIX
STOOLS/HOUR AND
VOMITING

LESS THAN SIX STOOLS/HOUR,
MINIMAL VOMITING, MILD
DEHYDRATION

HOSPITALIZE FOR
IV FLUIDS, ANTIEMETICS,
DIPHENOXYLATE HCl

TREAT AT HOME WITH
BALANCED ELECTROLYTE
SOLUTIONS, DIPHENOXYLATE
HCl, BISMUTH PREPARATIONS

IDENTIFY
ORGANISM
IF POSSIBLE

POOR RESULTS

GOOD
RESULTS

IDENTIFY
ORGANISM IF
POSSIBLE, ADMIT
TO HOSPITAL

OBSERVE

GAUCHER'S DISEASE

1. Confirm diagnosis with liver and bone marrow biopsy, enzyme assay, x-rays, and MRI.
2. No therapy is necessary in most patients.
3. Partial or total splenectomy. Should have pneumococcal vaccination prior to splenectomy.
4. Administer aglucerase enzyme replacement therapy in severe cases. Cost may be prohibitive.

GIARDIASIS

1. Confirm diagnosis by stools for ovum and parasites and *Giardia* antigen.
2. Treat with metronidazole 250 mg t.i.d. for 5 days.
3. Alternate therapy is quinacrine 100 mg b.i.d. for 5 days.
4. Combined therapy may be utilized in refractory cases.

GILBERT'S DISEASE

1. Confirm diagnosis with liver function tests.
2. No therapy is necessary.

GINGIVITIS

1. Confirm diagnosis by clinical examination and dental consult.
2. Conservative measures include daily brushing of teeth, flossing, and mouth rinses.
3. Refer to a dental hygienist for regular cleaning and plaque removal.
4. Antibiotic packing of deep pockets may be tried by a dentist in resistive cases.
5. Refer to a periodontist for gingivectomy if medical treatment fails.

GLANDERS

1. Confirm diagnosis with culture of exudates and serological tests.
2. Surgical drainage of abscessed lesions.
3. Treat with ceftazidime 750–1000 mg q.12h. IM or IV for 30 days. Alternatively, patient may be given trimethoprim-sulfamethoxazole combinations twice daily for 30 days.

GLANZMANN'S DISEASE

1. Confirm diagnosis with coagulation studies, CBC, platelet count, and clot retraction tests.
2. Treat only significant hemorrhage and blood loss with platelet transfusions. Consult a hematologist.

GLAUCOMA

1. Confirm diagnosis with tonometry or ophthalmology consult.
2. *Primary open-angle glaucoma:*
   a. Treat with topical pharmacologic agents (such as timolol solution 0.25% b.i.d.). Ophthalmology consult is wise before treatment.
   b. Argon laser trabeculoplasty if above unsatisfactory.
   c. Trabeculectomy.
3. *Primary angle-closure glaucoma:* This is a medical emergency, and the patient should be referred to an ophthalmologist immediately.

GLOMERULONEPHRITIS

1. Confirm diagnosis by urinalysis, ASO titer, C3 complement levels, and renal biopsy. Consult a nephrologist.
2. *Acute glomerulonephritis:*
   a. Treat underlying streptococcal or other bacterial infection with antibiotics.
   b. Treat mild hypertension and fluid retention with salt restriction and loop diuretics.
   c. Treat severe hypertension with vasodilator drugs such as hydralazine, nifedipine, or diazoxide.
   d. Treat acute renal failure with ion exchange resins or dialysis (see Acute Renal Failure, page 410).
3. *Rapidly progressive glomerulonephritis:*
   a. Consult a nephrologist.
   b. Corticosteroids and cytotoxic agents may be necessary but often unsuccessful.
   c. Plasmapheresis may be tried.
   d. Renal dialysis and renal transplant need to be considered.
4. Chronic glomerulonephritis: Treatment for this disorder is the same as for chronic renal failure (see page 412).

GLYCOGEN STORAGE DISEASE

1. Confirm diagnosis with blood chemistries, liver and muscle biopsy, and enzyme assay of tissue samples.
2. Type Ia (von Gierke's disease) and type Ib can be treated with frequent daytime and nighttime feedings, cornstarch, and restriction of sucrose and lactose. Consult a dietician. Control uric acid level with allopurinol.
3. Type III and IV are also treated with frequent feedings and cornstarch, but the diet can contain more protein. Consult a dietician.
4. Type V and VII involve the muscles and are treated with glucose and fructose before exercise. Exercise should be avoided.
5. There is no effective treatment for type II and VI.

GOITER, DIFFUSE

1. Confirm diagnosis with free T_4, TSH, antithyroglobulin antibodies, RAI uptake and scan, and ultrasound.
2. *Simple nontoxic goiter:* Treat with levothyroxine 100–300 µg a day. If gland reduces in size, follow patient. If gland does not decrease in size, reevaluate diagnosis. Surgery is reserved for large goiters with obstructive symptoms or when carcinoma is suspected.
3. *Toxic multinodular goiter:* Bring patient to euthyroid state with antithyroid drugs (propylthiouracil, etc.), then give radioactive iodine. Consult a radiotherapist or endocrinologist. Surgery for resistant cases.
4. *Hashimoto's thyroiditis:*
   a. With hypothyroidism, treat with levothyroxine 100–300 µg/day. Monitor TSH.
   b. With hyperthyroidism, treat with antithyroid drugs until becomes euthyroid or hypothyroid.
5. *Graves' disease:* See Hyperthyroidism, page 225.

GOITER, DIFFUSE

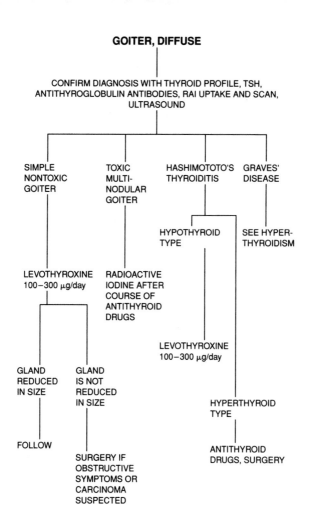

CONFIRM DIAGNOSIS WITH THYROID PROFILE, TSH, ANTITHYROGLOBULIN ANTIBODIES, RAI UPTAKE AND SCAN, ULTRASOUND

SIMPLE NONTOXIC GOITER

TOXIC MULTI-NODULAR GOITER

HASHIMOTOTO'S THYROIDITIS

GRAVES' DISEASE

HYPOTHYROID TYPE

SEE HYPER-THYROIDISM

LEVOTHYROXINE 100–300 µg/day

RADIOACTIVE IODINE AFTER COURSE OF ANTITHYROID DRUGS

LEVOTHYROXINE 100–300 µg/day

GLAND REDUCED IN SIZE

GLAND IS NOT REDUCED IN SIZE

HYPERTHYROID TYPE

FOLLOW

SURGERY IF OBSTRUCTIVE SYMPTOMS OR CARCINOMA SUSPECTED

ANTITHYROID DRUGS, SURGERY

GONORRHEA

1. Confirm diagnosis by smear, culture of exudate, blood cultures, and enzyme-linked immunosorbent assay (ELISA).
2. *Uncomplicated infections:* Treat with ceftriaxone 125 mg IM and follow with doxycycline 100 mg b.i.d. p.o. for 7 days. Recheck patient for treatment failure.
3. *Pelvic inflammatory disease:* Hospitalize and administer doxycycline 100 mg IV q.12h. plus cefotetan 2 gm q.12h. IV or cefoxitin 2 g q.12h. IV. Continue these drugs for 48 hours after clinical recovery and follow with oral doxycycline for a total of 14 days.
4. *Gonorrhea in pregnancy:* Administer ceftriaxone 125 mg IM and follow with erythromycin 500 mg q.i.d. for 7 days.
5. *Disseminated gonococcal infections (such as arthritis and endocarditis):* Hospitalize and treat with ceftriaxone 1 g/day IV for 7–14 days. Continue treatment longer if there is endocarditis or meningitis. Patients may be transferred to oral therapy (such as cefixime 400 mg b.i.d.) once clinical resolution is apparent for 48 hours.
6. Rapid identification of sexual partners is essential to prevent the spread of the disease and the reinfection of the cured patient.

GONORRHEA

CONFIRM DIAGNOSIS BY SMEAR, CULTURE OF EXUDATE OR
BLOOD, AND ENZYME-LINKED IMMUNOSORBENT ASSAY (ELISA)

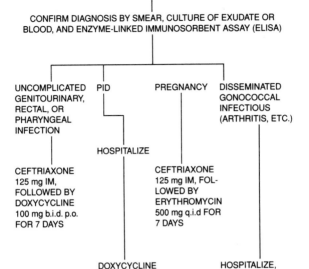

UNCOMPLICATED
GENITOURINARY,
RECTAL, OR
PHARYNGEAL
INFECTION

PID

PREGNANCY

DISSEMINATED
GONOCOCCAL
INFECTIOUS
(ARTHRITIS, ETC.)

HOSPITALIZE

CEFTRIAXONE
125 mg IM,
FOLLOWED BY
DOXYCYCLINE
100 mg b.i.d. p.o.
FOR 7 DAYS

CEFTRIAXONE
125 mg IM, FOL-
LOWED BY
ERYTHROMYCIN
500 mg q.i.d FOR
7 DAYS

DOXYCYCLINE
100 mg IV q. 12 h.
PLUS
CEFOTETAN 2 gm
q. 12 h IV

HOSPITALIZE,
CEFTRIAXONE
1 gm/day IV FOR
7–10 DAYS

GOODPASTURE'S DISEASE

1. Confirm the diagnosis by immunoassay of circulating antibodies to glycopeptide antigens related to basement membrane collagen. Consult a nephrologist for renal biopsy if necessary.
2. Treat with plasma exchange therapy combined with intravenous methylprednisolone 1 g/day for three consecutive days, followed by 60 mg of prednisone daily for 4–6 weeks. After that, the prednisone is gradually tapered.
3. Cyclophosphamide 2 mg/kg daily may be administered concurrently with the corticosteroids. Consult an oncologist or a rheumatologist.
4. If the disease progresses, renal dialysis or renal transplant may be necessary. Consult a nephrologist.

GOUT

1. Confirm diagnosis by blood uric acid levels, synovial fluid analysis, and response to colchicine.
2. *Acute gouty arthritis:* Administer colchicine 0.6 mg hourly until symptoms subside or gastrointestinal symptoms develop. Then give a maintenance dose of colchicine 0.6 mg b.i.d. to q.i.d. Alternatively, indomethacin 50 mg q.i.d. or sulindac 200 mg b.i.d. may be given. Intra-articular corticosteroids (such as triamcinolone 20 mg and 2–4 cc of 1–2% lidocaine) may be given.
3. *Asymptomatic hyperuricemia:* No treatment is necessary unless the patient is about to undergo cancer chemotherapy.
4. *Chronic gouty arthritis:* Eliminate uric acid deposits and hyperuricemia with allopurinol 300 mg/day in single dose or probenecid 250 mg b.i.d. Probenecid may be increased to 3 g/day if necessary. Alternatively, sulfinpyrazone 50 mg b.i.d. may be given. That dose may be increased to 400 mg/day if necessary.

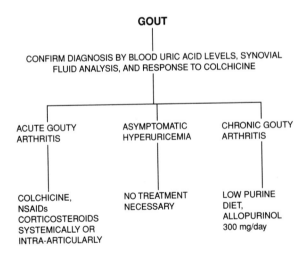

GOUT

CONFIRM DIAGNOSIS BY BLOOD URIC ACID LEVELS, SYNOVIAL FLUID ANALYSIS, AND RESPONSE TO COLCHICINE

ACUTE GOUTY ARTHRITIS

ASYMPTOMATIC HYPERURICEMIA

CHRONIC GOUTY ARTHRITIS

COLCHICINE, NSAIDs CORTICOSTEROIDS SYSTEMICALLY OR INTRA-ARTICULARLY

NO TREATMENT NECESSARY

LOW PURINE DIET, ALLOPURINOL 300 mg/day

GRANULOMA INGUINALE

1. Confirm diagnosis with Giemsa or Wright's stain of scrapings from lesion or biopsy.
2. Treat with tetracycline 500 mg q.i.d. p.o. for 14–21 days, or trimethoprim-sulfamethoxazole double strength (160 mg and 800 mg, respectively) twice daily for 14–21 days.
3. Identify sexual partners.

GUILLAIN–BARRÉ SYNDROME

1. Confirm diagnosis by spinal fluid analysis, electromyography, and nerve conduction studies. Consult a neurologist.
2. *Acute demyelinating neuropathy:*
   a. Hospitalize for respiratory, cardiovascular, and general supportive care. Respiratory paralysis is a very real concern.
   b. Try plasmapheresis.
   c. High-dose immunoglobulin therapy (2 g per kilogram of body weight over a 5-day period) may be just as effective as plasmapheresis.
   d. Corticosteroids are of no proven value but may be tried.
3. *Chronic demyelinating neuropathy:*
   a. Corticosteroids may be tried first, such as prednisone 60–80 mg/day over 4–6 weeks and gradually tapering.
   b. Plasmapheresis.
   c. High-dose immunoglobulin therapy as detailed above.

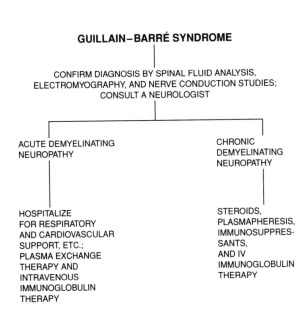

GUILLAIN–BARRÉ SYNDROME

CONFIRM DIAGNOSIS BY SPINAL FLUID ANALYSIS, ELECTROMYOGRAPHY, AND NERVE CONDUCTION STUDIES; CONSULT A NEUROLOGIST

ACUTE DEMYELINATING NEUROPATHY

CHRONIC DEMYELINATING NEUROPATHY

HOSPITALIZE FOR RESPIRATORY AND CARDIOVASCULAR SUPPORT, ETC.; PLASMA EXCHANGE THERAPY AND INTRAVENOUS IMMUNOGLOBULIN THERAPY

STEROIDS, PLASMAPHERESIS, IMMUNOSUPPRESSANTS, AND IV IMMUNOGLOBULIN THERAPY

HARTNUP DISEASE

1. Confirm diagnosis by urinalysis for amino acids.
2. Treat with niacinamide 40–200 mg/day and a high-protein diet.
3. The prognosis is good as the disease improves with age.

HEAD INJURY

1. Confirm type of injury with skull x-ray and CT scan. MRI is more useful later.
2. *Concussion;*
   a. Mild to moderate: Observation, symptomatic treatment.
   b. Moderate to severe: Hospitalize for observation and supportive care. Look for post-traumatic epilepsy.
3. *Skull fracture (consult a neurosurgeon):*
   a. Nondepressed: Observation.
   b. Depressed: Surgery if depressed more than 5 mm.
4. *Epidural hematoma:*
   a. Neurosurgical consultation.
   b. Surgery as indicated.
5. *Subdural hematoma:*
   a. Neurosurgical consultation.
   b. Surgery as indicated.
6. Intracerebral hematoma:
   a. Small: Observe. May consult a neurosurgeon.
   b. Large: Surgery.
7. *Increased intracranial pressure:* ICP pressure monitoring, mannitol, diuretics, and hyperventilation.
8. *Prognosis:* Subdural and epidural hematomas can be rapidly fatal. Morbidity is high with subdural hematomas.

HEAD INJURY

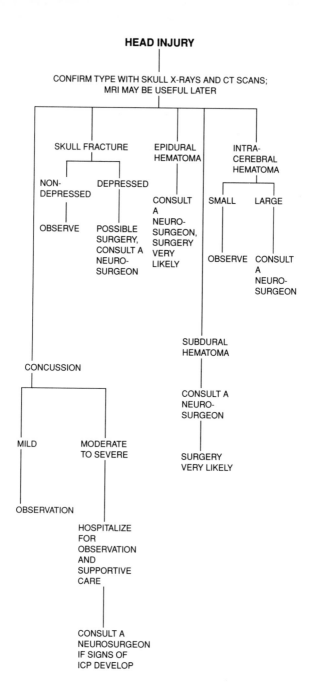

CONFIRM TYPE WITH SKULL X-RAYS AND CT SCANS;
MRI MAY BE USEFUL LATER

SKULL FRACTURE

EPIDURAL HEMATOMA

INTRA-CEREBRAL HEMATOMA

NON-DEPRESSED

DEPRESSED

OBSERVE

POSSIBLE SURGERY, CONSULT A NEURO-SURGEON

CONSULT A NEURO-SURGEON, SURGERY VERY LIKELY

SMALL

LARGE

OBSERVE

CONSULT A NEURO-SURGEON

CONCUSSION

SUBDURAL HEMATOMA

CONSULT A NEURO-SURGEON

MILD

MODERATE TO SEVERE

SURGERY VERY LIKELY

OBSERVATION

HOSPITALIZE FOR OBSERVATION AND SUPPORTIVE CARE

CONSULT A NEUROSURGEON IF SIGNS OF ICP DEVELOP

HEART FAILURE

1. Confirm diagnosis with EKG, chest x-ray, spirometry, venous pressure and circulation time, and echocardiography. If necessary, consult a cardiologist to assist in the diagnosis and determining the cause.

2. *Acute onset:* Hospitalize for complete bed rest, continuous oxygen therapy, IV diuretics (furosemide, etc.), and vasodilators. Consult a cardiologist to advise on the use of nitroprusside, digoxin, and sympathomimetic amines. Consider phlebotomy in refractory cases. Monitor intake and output. Restrict fluid intake to 1000 cc or less each day.

3. *Gradual onset:*
   a. With atrial fibrillation, consider digoxin. Loading dose of 0.25 mg q.i.d., followed by 0.125–0.25 mg/day. Monitor blood levels. If symptoms persist, add diuretics (furosemide 20–80 mg/day) and/or ACE inhibitors (enalapril 20 mg/day or lisinopril 10 mg/day). If resolution is still not apparent, consult a cardiologist.
   b. Without atrial fibrillation: Try diuretics (furosemide 20–80 mg/day) first. If unsuccessful, add ACE inhibitors (enalapril 20 mg/day or lisinopril 10 mg/day). If symptoms persist, consult a cardiologist for advice about vasodilators and digoxin use.

4. Consider cardiovascular surgery and heart transplant with the aid of a cardiologist or cardiovascular surgeon.

HEART FAILURE

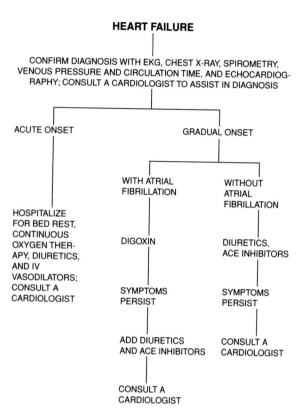

CONFIRM DIAGNOSIS WITH EKG, CHEST X-RAY, SPIROMETRY, VENOUS PRESSURE AND CIRCULATION TIME, AND ECHOCARDIOGRAPHY; CONSULT A CARDIOLOGIST TO ASSIST IN DIAGNOSIS

ACUTE ONSET

GRADUAL ONSET

WITH ATRIAL FIBRILLATION

WITHOUT ATRIAL FIBRILLATION

HOSPITALIZE FOR BED REST, CONTINUOUS OXYGEN THERAPY, DIURETICS, AND IV VASODILATORS; CONSULT A CARDIOLOGIST

DIGOXIN

DIURETICS, ACE INHIBITORS

SYMPTOMS PERSIST

SYMPTOMS PERSIST

ADD DIURETICS AND ACE INHIBITORS

CONSULT A CARDIOLOGIST

CONSULT A CARDIOLOGIST

HEAT-RELATED DISORDERS

1. Confirm diagnosis by body temperature and by presence or absence of sweat.
2. *Heat exhaustion:* Treat by placing in a cool environment in recumbent position. Start IV or oral hypotonic saline solutions.
3. *Heat stroke:* Hospitalize for intensive care. Remove clothing and start continuous spray of cool water, and use IV hypotonic saline solutions judiciously because patient may only require 1000–1500 cc of replacement fluids.
4. If complications develop (renal, cardiovascular, neurological, etc.), consult an appropriate specialist.

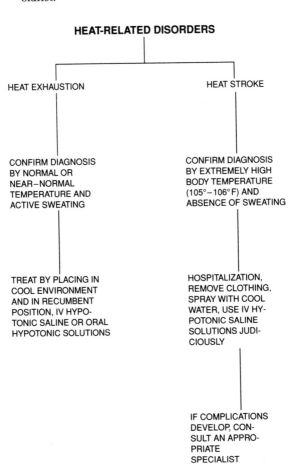

HEAT-RELATED DISORDERS

HEAT EXHAUSTION

CONFIRM DIAGNOSIS BY NORMAL OR NEAR-NORMAL TEMPERATURE AND ACTIVE SWEATING

TREAT BY PLACING IN COOL ENVIRONMENT AND IN RECUMBENT POSITION, IV HYPOTONIC SALINE OR ORAL HYPOTONIC SOLUTIONS

HEAT STROKE

CONFIRM DIAGNOSIS BY EXTREMELY HIGH BODY TEMPERATURE (105°–106° F) AND ABSENCE OF SWEATING

HOSPITALIZATION, REMOVE CLOTHING, SPRAY WITH COOL WATER, USE IV HYPOTONIC SALINE SOLUTIONS JUDICIOUSLY

IF COMPLICATIONS DEVELOP, CONSULT AN APPROPRIATE SPECIALIST

HEMANGIOBLASTOMA

1. Confirm diagnosis with CT scans, MRI, or vertebral angiography.
2. Consult a neurosurgeon for resection.
3. *Prognosis:* Over 75% of the patients are alive and functioning well up to 20 years after surgery. Tumor may recur if only partially removed.

HEMIFACIAL SPASM

1. Confirm diagnosis by clinical evaluation.
2. Give a trial of anticonvulsant therapy (phenytoin 300–600 mg/day, carbamazepine 400–1200 mg/day, or clonazepam 0.5–5 mg/day in divided doses).
3. Inject botulinum toxin in affected muscles. Consult a neurologist.
4. Consult a neurosurgeon for exploration of facial nerve in the posterior fossa with microvascular decompression.

HEMOCHROMATOSIS

1. Confirm diagnosis with serum iron, iron-binding capacity, ferritin, and liver biopsy.
2. Treat with intermittent phlebotomy. May need to be weekly for up to 2–3 years. Consult a hematologist for guidance.
3. Observe for development of hepatic carcinoma, diabetes, or heart failure.

HEMOGLOBIN C DISEASE

1. Confirm diagnosis by CBC, blood smear, red cell fragility, and hemoglobin electrophoresis.
2. Treatment is supportive. There is no specific therapy for this disease.

HEMOLYTIC ANEMIA, ACQUIRED

1. Confirm diagnosis by CBC, red cell fragility test, and direct and indirect Coombs' tests.
2. Consult a hematologist to look for cause and assist in therapy.
3. If there is only mild hemolysis, do nothing.
4. First-line therapy is prednisone 1 mg/kg daily 4–8 weeks and taper.
5. Transfusions for patients with significant anemia.
6. If corticosteroids are ineffective, a splenectomy may be necessary. Consult a hematologist. Patients should be given pneumococcal vaccine.
7. If both corticosteroids and splenectomy are ineffective, immunosuppressant drugs should be tried (i.e., cyclophosphamide or azathioprine). Consult an oncologist for guidance.

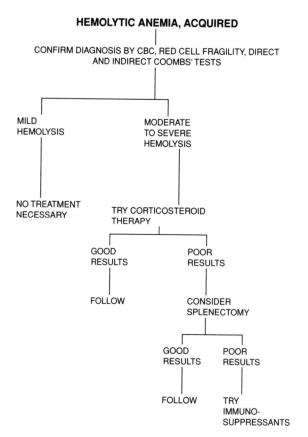

HEMOLYTIC ANEMIA, ACQUIRED

CONFIRM DIAGNOSIS BY CBC, RED CELL FRAGILITY, DIRECT AND INDIRECT COOMBS' TESTS

MILD HEMOLYSIS — NO TREATMENT NECESSARY

MODERATE TO SEVERE HEMOLYSIS — TRY CORTICOSTEROID THERAPY

GOOD RESULTS — FOLLOW

POOR RESULTS — CONSIDER SPLENECTOMY

GOOD RESULTS — FOLLOW

POOR RESULTS — TRY IMMUNO-SUPPRESSANTS

HEMOPHILIA

1. Confirm diagnosis with coagulation time, prothrombin time, partial thromboplastin time, and assays for Factors VIII, IX, and XI.
2. *Factor VIII deficiency:* Cryoprecipitate, Factor VIII concentrate. Consult a hematologist. May use fresh-frozen plasma while waiting for above.
3. *Factor IX deficiency:* Fresh-frozen plasma or plasma fraction enriched in prothrombin complex proteins. Consult a hematologist.
4. *Factor XI deficiency:* Fresh-frozen plasma. Consult a hematologist.

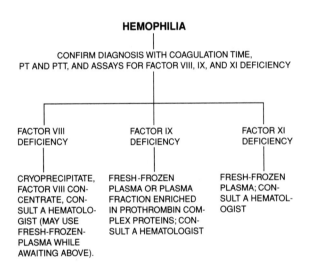

HEMOPHILIA

CONFIRM DIAGNOSIS WITH COAGULATION TIME,
PT AND PTT, AND ASSAYS FOR FACTOR VIII, IX, AND XI DEFICIENCY

FACTOR VIII DEFICIENCY	FACTOR IX DEFICIENCY	FACTOR XI DEFICIENCY
CRYOPRECIPITATE, FACTOR VIII CONCENTRATE, CONSULT A HEMATOLOGIST (MAY USE FRESH-FROZEN-PLASMA WHILE AWAITING ABOVE).	FRESH-FROZEN PLASMA OR PLASMA FRACTION ENRICHED IN PROTHROMBIN COMPLEX PROTEINS; CONSULT A HEMATOLOGIST	FRESH-FROZEN PLASMA; CONSULT A HEMATOLOGIST

HEMORRHAGIC FEVER

1. This disorder is associated with numerous arboviruses-arenaviruses, including yellow fever, dengue, Omsk hemorrhagic fever, and Congo-Crimean hemorrhagic fever.
2. Confirm diagnosis by clinical evaluation and leukopenia and specific serologic tests when available. Viral isolation may be possible.
3. Treatment is supportive. There is no specific therapy.

HEMORRHOIDS

1. Confirm diagnosis by digital examination, anoscopy, or proctoscopy. If they are chronically bleeding, colonoscopy should be done to be sure there is no other site of bleeding (colon carcinoma).
2. *External hemorrhoids:*
   a. Thrombosed: Incision and drainage.
   b. Not thrombosed: Conservative therapy with sitz baths, stool softeners, suppositories, or gentian violet 1% applied after each BM.
   c. If they persist, consider surgery.
3. *Internal hemorrhoids:*
   a. Permanent prolapse: Surgery.
   b. Intermittent prolapse or bleeding: Try banding or sclerotherapy.
   c. If they persist, call a proctologist.

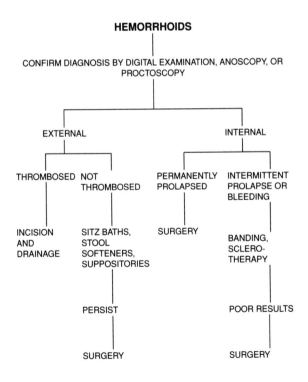

HEPATITIS, TOXIC

1. Confirm diagnosis by history of drug ingestion, liver function tests, negative studies for viral hepatitis, and liver biopsy.
2. Withdrawal of the drug is usually all that is necessary.
3. In persistent cases, consult a gastroenterologist or a hepatologist.
4. Cholestyramine may be used to relieve itching.
5. In cases of acetaminophen toxicity, cysteine or N-acetylcysteine may reduce hepatic necrosis. Consult a hepatologist.

HEPATITIS, VIRAL

1. Confirm diagnosis with liver function tests and serologic tests for A, B, C, and D forms.
2. *Acute hepatitis*:
   a. Mild to moderate: May treat at home with isolation from rest of family and high-calorie diet.
   b. Severe: Hospitalize, low-protein diet, lactulose, neomycin for bowel sterilization, and consult a gastroenterologist.
3. *Chronic hepatitis:*
   a. Chronic active: Corticosteroids usually no benefit. Consider a transplant.
   b. Autoimmune type: Corticosteroids effective in many cases.
   c. Postnecrotic cirrhosis: Treat conservatively; observe for complications and treat with help of a gastroenterologist.

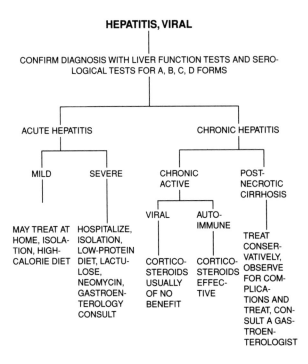

HEPATITIS, VIRAL

CONFIRM DIAGNOSIS WITH LIVER FUNCTION TESTS AND SEROLOGICAL TESTS FOR A, B, C, D FORMS

ACUTE HEPATITIS

CHRONIC HEPATITIS

MILD — MAY TREAT AT HOME, ISOLATION, HIGH-CALORIE DIET

SEVERE — HOSPITALIZE, ISOLATION, LOW-PROTEIN DIET, LACTULOSE, NEOMYCIN, GASTROENTEROLOGY CONSULT

CHRONIC ACTIVE

POSTNECROTIC CIRRHOSIS — TREAT CONSERVATIVELY, OBSERVE FOR COMPLICATIONS AND TREAT, CONSULT A GASTROENTEROLOGIST

VIRAL — CORTICOSTEROIDS USUALLY OF NO BENEFIT

AUTOIMMUNE — CORTICOSTEROIDS EFFECTIVE

HEPATOLENTICULAR DEGENERATION

1. Confirm the diagnosis by serum and urine copper, serum ceruloplasmin level, and liver biopsy.
2. Administer penicillamine 1 g/day divided into three doses, given 30 minutes before meals.
3. Observe the hypersensitivity reactions. If they occur, withdraw the drug and restart the drug with daily doses of prednisone (20 mg/day).
4. Lifelong therapy is required.
5. Follow with urinary copper determinations and liver function testing. A hepatologist should be consulted.

HEPATOMA

1. Confirm diagnosis with liver function tests, alpha-fetoprotein, CT scans, and liver biopsy.
2. Consult a surgeon for possible resection if tumor is confined to one lobe.
3. Consult an oncologist for evaluation for chemotherapy, but results have been disappointing.
4. For severe pain, consider chemoembolization.
5. *Prognosis:* Poor for survival beyond 1 year unless resection is feasible.

HEREDITARY ATAXIAS

1. Confirm diagnosis by clinical evaluation and neurologic consult.
2. No specific treatment is available.
3. Consult an orthopedic surgeon for treatment of contractures and foot deformities.
4. Prevention by genetic counseling.

HEREDITARY ELLIPTOCYTOSIS

1. Confirm diagnosis with CBC, blood sugar, serum haptoglobins, and red cell survival times.
2. Treatment is conservative because splenectomy is rarely required. Consult a hematologist.

HEREDITARY SPHEROCYTOSIS

1. Confirm diagnosis by family history, CBC, blood sugar, red cell fragility, and red cell survival times.
2. Consult a hematologist for evaluation for splenectomy. Pneumococcal vaccine should be given prior to splenectomy.
3. Evaluate adults for gallstones.

HERNIATED DISK, CERVICAL

1. Confirm diagnosis by MRI, combined CT scan and myelography, electromyography, or dermatomal somatosensory evoked potentials (DSEP).
2. *Quadriplegia:* Consult a neurosurgeon for immediate laminectomy.
3. No quadriplegia or paraplegia, but radiculopathy with upper extremity weakness: Neurosurgical evaluation before beginning conservative treatment.
3. No quadriplegia or paraplegia and no significant upper extremity weakness, but radiculopathy and neck pain: Begin conservative treatment with bed rest, traction, cervical collar, muscle relaxant, NSAIDs, and analgesics for 1–2 weeks.
4. *Conservative therapy ineffective:* Consult a neurologist or a neurosurgeon.
5. *Conservative therapy effective:* Follow up with physiotherapy and exercises.

Drugs and Dosages

1. *Muscle relaxants:*
   a. Carisoprodol 350 mg t.i.d.
   b. Cyclobenzaprine HCl 10–20 mg t.i.d.
   c. Chlorzoxazone 250–750 mg t.i.d. with Tylenol.
   d. Orphenadrine citrate 100 mg b.i.d.
2. *NSAIDs:*
   a. Naproxen 250–500 mg t.i.d.
   b. Ibuprofen 400–800 mg t.i.d.
   c. Sulindac 150–200 mg b.i.d.
   d. Piroxicam 20 mg/day.
3. *Analgesics:*
   a. Codeine (15–60 mg) and acetaminophen (325–650 mg) q.4–6h. p.r.n.
   b. Hydrocodone (5–10 mg) and acetaminophen (325–650 mg) q.4–6h. p.r.n.

HERNIATED DISK, CERVICAL

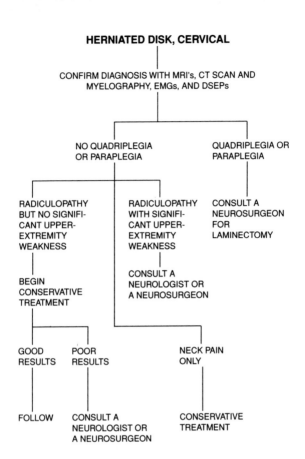

CONFIRM DIAGNOSIS WITH MRI's, CT SCAN AND MYELOGRAPHY, EMGs, AND DSEPs

NO QUADRIPLEGIA OR PARAPLEGIA

QUADRIPLEGIA OR PARAPLEGIA

RADICULOPATHY BUT NO SIGNIFICANT UPPER-EXTREMITY WEAKNESS

RADICULOPATHY WITH SIGNIFICANT UPPER-EXTREMITY WEAKNESS

CONSULT A NEUROSURGEON FOR LAMINECTOMY

BEGIN CONSERVATIVE TREATMENT

CONSULT A NEUROLOGIST OR A NEUROSURGEON

GOOD RESULTS

POOR RESULTS

NECK PAIN ONLY

FOLLOW

CONSULT A NEUROLOGIST OR A NEUROSURGEON

CONSERVATIVE TREATMENT

HERNIATED DISK, LUMBAR

1. Confirm diagnosis by MRI, CT scans, combined CT scan and myelography, EMG (electromyography), or DSEP (dermatomal somatosensory evoked potential study).
2. Patient has urinary retention, atrophy, paraplegia, or monoplegia (foot drop, etc.): Consult a neurosurgeon for laminectomy.
3. Patient has no urinary retention, atrophy, paraplegia, or monoplegia: Treat conservatively with bed rest, muscle relaxants, NSAIDs, analgesics, epidural blocks, and physiotherapy. Consider chiropractic care.
4. *Poor response to conservative therapy:*
   a. Patient has mild to moderate pain but no neurologic deficit: Continue physiotherapy and prescribe exercise and job retraining, if necessary.
   b. Patient has either severe pain or significant neurologic deficit: Neurological or neurosurgical consult.

Drugs: See page 205.

HERNIATED DISK, LUMBAR

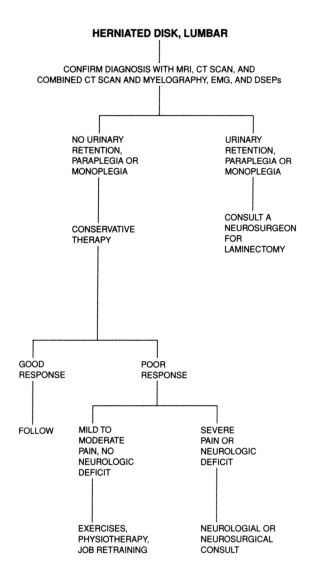

CONFIRM DIAGNOSIS WITH MRI, CT SCAN, AND
COMBINED CT SCAN AND MYELOGRAPHY, EMG, AND DSEPs

NO URINARY RETENTION, PARAPLEGIA OR MONOPLEGIA

URINARY RETENTION, PARAPLEGIA OR MONOPLEGIA

CONSULT A NEUROSURGEON FOR LAMINECTOMY

CONSERVATIVE THERAPY

GOOD RESPONSE

POOR RESPONSE

FOLLOW

MILD TO MODERATE PAIN, NO NEUROLOGIC DEFICIT

SEVERE PAIN OR NEUROLOGIC DEFICIT

EXERCISES, PHYSIOTHERAPY, JOB RETRAINING

NEUROLOGIAL OR NEUROSURGICAL CONSULT

HERPANGINA

1. Confirm diagnosis by history and physical and oral surgical consult.
2. No specific therapy indicated because healing usually occurs without treatment.

HERPES SIMPLEX

1. Confirm diagnosis by clinical evaluation.
2. *Primary infection:* Treat with acyclovir capsules 200 mg five times a day for 7 days.
3. *Recurrent infection:* Spontaneous healing frequently occurs, but acyclovir 200 mg five times a day for 7 days may be administered for persistent cases. A newer compound, volacyclovir HCL can be conveniently given twice daily at a 500 mg dose for only 5 days. Evaluate patient's immune system.
4. *Disseminated infections:* Acyclovir intravenously 5–10 mg/kg q.8h. is indicated. Consult an infectious disease specialist. Look for HIV infection.

HERPES ZOSTER

1. Confirm diagnosis by clinical evaluation, Tancz test, serology, and animal inoculation.
2. Treat with acyclovir 800 mg five times a day for 7–10 days. A newer compound, volacyclovir HCL can be given 1000 mg twice daily for 7 days.
3. Postherpetic neuralgia may be treated with tricyclic antidepressants (such as amitriptyline 25–150 mg daily) or nerve blocks or by providing the patient with a portable TENS unit.
4. *Disseminated infections in immunocompromised hosts:* Acyclovir intravenously 5–10 mg/kg q.8h. Consult an infectious disease specialist.

HIDRADENITIS SUPPURATIVA

1. Confirm diagnosis with clinical evaluation and cultures of exudates.
2. Consult a surgeon for I&D.
3. Administer oral antistaphylococcus antibiotics such as dicloxacillin or cloxacillin 500 mg q.i.d. for 7–10 days.

HIRSCHSPRUNG'S DISEASE

1. Confirm diagnosis by physical, barium enema, and surgical biopsy of the colon under anesthesia.
2. Consult a surgeon for surgical bypass of the aganglionic segment of bowel.

HISTAMINE CEPHALALGIA

1. Confirm diagnosis by clinical evaluation, histamine test, and response to sumatriptan.
2. *Acute attack:* Sumatriptan 6 mg subcutaneously is preferred. Dihydroergotamine IM or IV may also be effective. Oxygen and parenteral narcotics may be necessary if the above treatment fails.
3. *Prophylaxis:*
   a. Administer prednisone 1 mg/kg daily for 7–10 days and gradually taper.
   b. If prednisone is ineffective, try methysergide 2–4 mg t.i.d. until attacks are prevented for 10–14 days.
   c. If above treatment is ineffective, consult a neurologist.

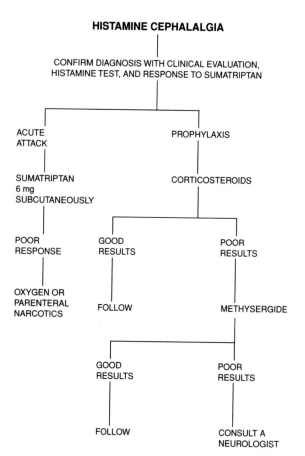

HISTAMINE CEPHALALGIA

CONFIRM DIAGNOSIS WITH CLINICAL EVALUATION, HISTAMINE TEST, AND RESPONSE TO SUMATRIPTAN

ACUTE ATTACK

PROPHYLAXIS

SUMATRIPTAN 6 mg SUBCUTANEOUSLY

CORTICOSTEROIDS

POOR RESPONSE

GOOD RESULTS

POOR RESULTS

OXYGEN OR PARENTERAL NARCOTICS

FOLLOW

METHYSERGIDE

GOOD RESULTS

POOR RESULTS

FOLLOW

CONSULT A NEUROLOGIST

HISTIOCYTOSIS X

1. Confirm diagnosis with x-rays of the skull and long bones, bone scans, CT scans, and biopsy of the liver, spleen, or lymph nodes.
2. Corticosteroids and immunosuppressant agents may be tried. Consult an oncologist. Radiotherapy may be tried.
3. Diabetes insipidus is treated with Pitressin therapy (see page 109).

HISTOPLASMOSIS

1. Confirm diagnosis with serological tests, sputum culture, and skin tests.
2. *Acute respiratory histoplasmosis:* Usually no treatment necessary.
3. *Disseminated or chronic pulmonary histoplasmosis:*
   a. Ketoconazole 400 mg/day. If response is not adequate after 1 month, increase dose to 600–800 mg/day. Continue therapy for 6–12 months.
   b. Alternative drug is itraconazole 200 mg once or twice a day.
   c. In AIDS patients, consult an infectious disease specialist for use of amphotericin B.

HOOKWORM DISEASE

1. Confirm diagnosis by stool for ovum and parasites.
2. Treat with mebendazole 100 mg b.i.d. for 3 days or single dose of pyrantel pamoate 10 mg/kg.
3. Treat anemia with oral iron, such as ferrous sulfate 300 mg t.i.d.

HUNTINGTON'S CHOREA

1. Confirm diagnosis by family history and neurologic examination. Consult a neurologist.
2. Treatment is symptomatic with dopamine antagonists such as haloperidol 0.5–2.0 mg t.i.d. or
   tetrabenazine 25–50 mg t.i.d. Consult a neurologist.
3. Prevention by genetic screening and counseling.

HURLER'S SYNDROME

1. Confirm diagnosis by clinical evaluation, urine acid mucopolysaccharides, and determination of alpha-L-iduronidase in cultured skin fibroblasts and leukocytes.
2. No specific treatment is available.

HYDROCEPHALUS

1. Confirm diagnosis by MRI or CT scans and by lumbar isotope cisternography.
2. Consult a neurosurgeon for treatment by ventriculocisternal shunting, ventriculopleural shunting, or other shunt procedure.
3. *Prognosis:* In infantile hydrocephalus there is only a 50% survival after 15 years of age. If normal-pressure hydrocephalus is discovered early, as many as 60% of patients improve.

HYPERNEPHROMA

1. Confirm diagnosis by intravenous pyelography, nephrotomography, ultrasonography, or CT scan. Exploratory surgery may occasionally be necessary.
2. Consult a urologist and an oncologist for evaluation and staging. If there are no metastases, radical nephrectomy may be performed. If there are multiple metastases, chemotherapy is used. If there are isolated metastases, nodulectomy may be tried.

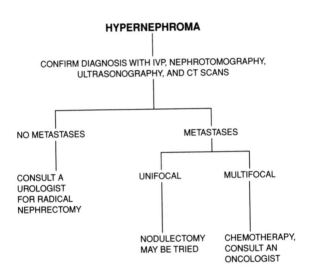

HYPERNEPHROMA

CONFIRM DIAGNOSIS WITH IVP, NEPHROTOMOGRAPHY, ULTRASONOGRAPHY, AND CT SCANS

NO METASTASES

CONSULT A UROLOGIST FOR RADICAL NEPHRECTOMY

METASTASES

UNIFOCAL

NODULECTOMY MAY BE TRIED

MULTIFOCAL

CHEMOTHERAPY, CONSULT AN ONCOLOGIST

HYPERPARATHYROIDISM

1. Confirm diagnosis by consistently elevated serum calcium and parathyroid hormone (PTH) immunoassay.
2. *Uncomplicated:*
   a. If the patient is young, surgery is advisable.
   b. If the patient is old (i.e., over 50), it may be wise to try medical treatment and follow the patient, observing for complications. Postmenopausal women may be treated with estrogen to lower the serum calcium and retard bone demineralization. Hydration alone will often lower the serum calcium. Consult an endocrinologist.
3. *Complicated:* If there is evidence of kidney stones or osteitis fibrosa cystica, surgery is indicated.
4. Follow postoperatively for the development of hypoparathyroidism.

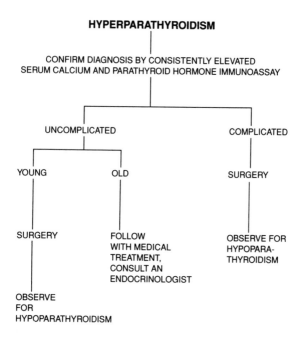

HYPERPARATHYROIDISM

CONFIRM DIAGNOSIS BY CONSISTENTLY ELEVATED
SERUM CALCIUM AND PARATHYROID HORMONE IMMUNOASSAY

UNCOMPLICATED

COMPLICATED

YOUNG

OLD

SURGERY

SURGERY

FOLLOW
WITH MEDICAL
TREATMENT,
CONSULT AN
ENDOCRINOLOGIST

OBSERVE FOR
HYPOPARA-
THYROIDISM

OBSERVE
FOR
HYPOPARATHYROIDISM

HYPERSENSITIVITY PNEUMONITIS

1. Confirm diagnosis by history, chest x-ray, pulmonary function tests, and immune response to the offending agent.
2. Many cases of acute exposure subside spontaneously with supportive care (oxygen, etc.).
3. If case is severe or fails to respond to supportive care, give 150 mg of hydrocortisone sodium succinate IV q.6h. Once there is improvement, patient may be given oral corticosteroids (prednisone 60 mg/day and gradually tapering over a 7- to 28-day period).
4. Remove patient from environmental exposure of the offending agent or alter the environment to prevent subsequent attacks and chronic form of the disease. For example, 1% propionic acid has been used on hay piles to reduce the growth of thermophilic organisms and control farmer's lung.
5. In chronic forms of the disease, strict avoidance of the offending agent must be applied, as well as long-term corticosteroids. Consult a pulmonologist.

HYPERSENSITIVITY VASCULITIS

1. Confirm diagnosis with CBC, ESR, and biopsy of skin.
2. Many cases resolve without treatment.
3. Treat underlying disease.
4. In persistent and severe cases, first give prednisone 1 mg/kg daily until therapeutic response and then gradually taper.
5. If corticosteroids are ineffective, give cyclophosphamide 2 mg/kg daily. Consult an oncologist for guidance.

HYPERTHYROIDISM

1. Confirm diagnosis with Free T_4 and radioactive iodine uptake (RAI) and scan.
2. *Toxic adenoma:* May treat with hemithyroidectomy or radioactive iodine 15–30 millicuries. Higher doses may be required.
3. *Graves' disease:*
   a. If there is severe cardiac disease, antithyroid drugs are the initial treatment. Once the patient has stabilized, radioactive iodine may be administered. If there is no cardiac disease, radioactive iodine is the treatment of choice. If there is a poor response to RAI, it should be repeated. Ultimately, surgery should be considered.
   b. During pregnancy: Consult an endocrinologist. Antithyroid drugs (propylthiouracil 100 mg q.i.d.) are recommended. If there is a poor response to these drugs, surgery should be considered. Once the pregnancy is over, the antithyroid drugs can be stopped and RAI administered.
   c. Children: Consult an endocrinologist. Antithyroid drugs may be tried. If these are unsuccessful, surgery should be considered.
   d. Thyroid storm: Hospitalize the patient in the intensive care unit and consult an endocrinologist. Treat with rehydration, propranolol IV 1–5 mg q.6h., and sodium iopodate 500 mg/day p.o. Carbamazole can be given, also, at the dose of 15 mg q.8h. Propranolol and sodium iopodate can be discontinued after 10–14 days, but antithyroid drugs should be continued until the decision is made on a long-range treatment plan.

HYPERTHYROIDISM

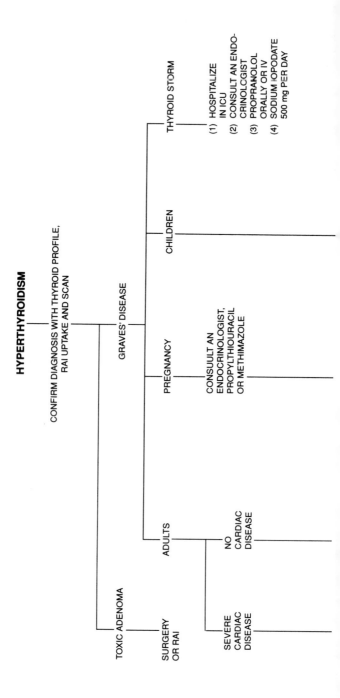

CONFIRM DIAGNOSIS WITH THYROID PROFILE, RAI UPTAKE AND SCAN

TOXIC ADENOMA

SURGERY OR RAI

GRAVES' DISEASE

ADULTS

SEVERE CARDIAC DISEASE

NO CARDIAC DISEASE

PREGNANCY

CONSUULT AN ENDOCRINOLOGIST, PROPYLTHIOURACIL OR METHIMAZOLE

CHILDREN

THYROID STORM

(1) HOSPITALIZE IN ICU
(2) CONSULT AN ENDO-CRINOLCGIST
(3) PROPRANOLOL ORALLY OR IV
(4) SODIUM IOPODATE 500 mg PER DAY

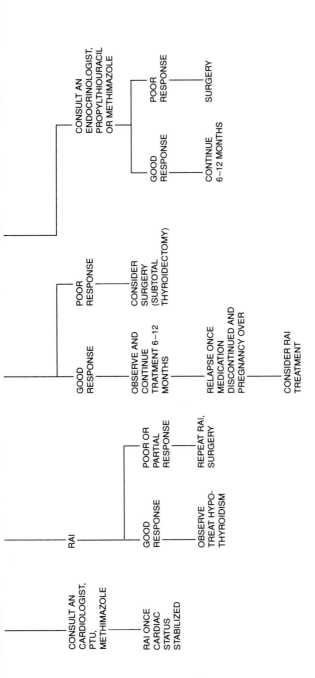

CONSULT AN CARDIOLOGIST, PTU, METHIMAZOLE

RAI ONCE CARDIAC STATUS STABILIZED

RAI

GOOD RESPONSE
OBSERVE TREAT HYPO-THYROIDISM

POOR OR PARTIAL RESPONSE
REPEAT RAI, SURGERY

GOOD RESPONSE
OBSERVE AND CONTINUE TRATMENT 6–12 MONTHS
RELAPSE ONCE MEDICATION DISCONTINUED AND PREGNANCY OVER
CONSIDER RAI TREATMENT

POOR RESPONSE
CONSIDER SURGERY (SUBTOTAL THYROIDECTOMY)

CONSULT AN ENDOCRINOLOGIST, PROPYLTHIOURACIL OR METHIMAZOLE

GOOD RESPONSE
CONTINUE 6–12 MONTHS

POOR RESPONSE
SURGERY

HYPOPARATHYROIDISM

1. Confirm diagnosis by serum calcium, phosphates, parathyroid hormone assay, and magnesium. Consult an endocrinlogist.
2. In chronic cases, initiate treatment with 2000–4000 mg of calcium and 1.25 mg of ergocalciferol t.i.d. May gradually increase the dose while monitoring serum calcium levels.
3. If hypercalciuria develops, treat with a thiazide diuretic.
4. If serum calcium levels cannot be brought to normal by the above program, switch to calcitriol therapy 0.5–3.0 μg/day.
5. Hypocalcemia due to surgically induced hypoparathyroidism (i.e., following a subtotal thyroidectomy) can be treated with 10 ml of calcium gluconate 10% solution IV and repeated until serum levels are normal. Following this, a continuous infusion can be administered (300–600 mg of calcium/day) until the patient can begin oral therapy. Oral therapy as outlined above should be started as soon as possible.
6. Evaluate for hypomagnesemia and treat.

HYPOPARATHYROIDISM

CONFIRM DIAGNOSIS BY SERUM CALCIUM, PHOSPHATES,
PARATHYROID HORMONE ASSAY, AND MAGNESIUM

ACUTE POSTSURGICAL

CALCIUM GLUCONATE
IV, FOLLOWED BY
ORAL CALCIUM
AND VITAMIN D
SUPPLEMENT

CHRONIC

CALCIUM AND
ERGOCALCIFEROL
IN INCREASING
DOES WHILE
MONITORING
SERUM CALCIUM

GOOD
RESPONSE

POOR
RESPONSE

FOLLOW

SWITCH TO
CALCITRIOL,
MONITOR SERUM
CALCIUM

HYPOPITUITARISM

1. Confirm diagnosis with free T_4, serum cortisol, serum growth hormone before and after insulin-induced hypoglycemia, metyrapone test, ACTH stimulation test, and serum FSH and LH. Consult an endocrinologist.
2. *Growth hormone deficiency:*
   a. Adults: No treatment.
   b. Children. Consult an endocrinologist.
3. *ACTH deficiency:*
   a. Administer cortisone acetate 25 mg in the morning and 12.5 mg before supper.
   b. Alternatively, give prednisone 5 mg in the morning and 2.5 mg before supper.
   c. Be sure to give additional corticosteroids during infections and before surgery (100 mg hydrocortisone sodium succinate before surgery and 50–100 mg IV q.6h. for 24–36 hours).
4. *TSH deficiency:*
   a. In younger patients, 100–125 µg of levothyroxine is the average dose.
   b. In older patients, 75–100 µg is the average dose.
   c. Monitor free T4 levels.
5. *Gonadotrophin deficiency:*
   a. In women with a uterus, estradiol 1–2 mg/day and medroxyprogesterone 2.5 mg/day may be given for 21–25 days per month.
   b. In women without a uterus, estradiol 1–2 mg/day for 25 days per month will be adequate.
   c. In men, testosterone cypionate 100–200 mg every 2 weeks deep IM is given.
6. *Prolactin deficiency:* Prolactin is not replaced.
7. *Antidiuretic hormone deficiency:* See Diabetes Insipidus, page 109.

HYPOPITUITARISM

CONFIRM DIAGNOSIS WITH
FREE T4, TSH, SERUM CORTISOL,
SERUM GROWTH HORMONE, ETC.

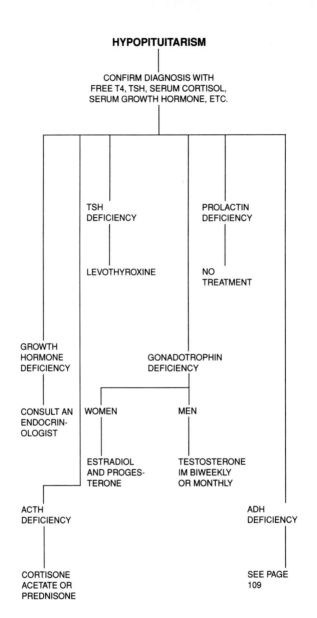

TSH
DEFICIENCY

LEVOTHYROXINE

PROLACTIN
DEFICIENCY

NO
TREATMENT

GROWTH
HORMONE
DEFICIENCY

GONADOTROPHIN
DEFICIENCY

CONSULT AN
ENDOCRIN-
OLOGIST

WOMEN

MEN

ESTRADIOL
AND PROGES-
TERONE

TESTOSTERONE
IM BIWEEKLY
OR MONTHLY

ACTH
DEFICIENCY

ADH
DEFICIENCY

CORTISONE
ACETATE OR
PREDNISONE

SEE PAGE
109

HYPOTHYROIDISM

1. Confirm diagnosis with free T_4 and serum TSH (sensitive assay).
2. *Uncomplicated hypothyroidism:* May begin levothyroxine at 50–100 µg/day and gradually increase until TSH is within normal range.
3. *Complicated hypothyroidism:*
   a. Heart disease: Begin therapy with lower doses such as 25 µg/day, increase 25 µg every 4 weeks. Usual maintenance dose is 100–125 µg/day. Consult a cardiologist.
   b. Pregnancy: An increased dose of levothyroxine may be needed. Monitor the TSH and bring it into normal range. Consult an endocrinologist.
   c. Myxedema coma: Admit to ICU; get endocrinology consult; sodium levothyroxine 500 µg IV; monitor T3 and T4 levels; administer hydrocortisone sodium succinate 100–300 µg/day.

HYPOTHYROIDISM

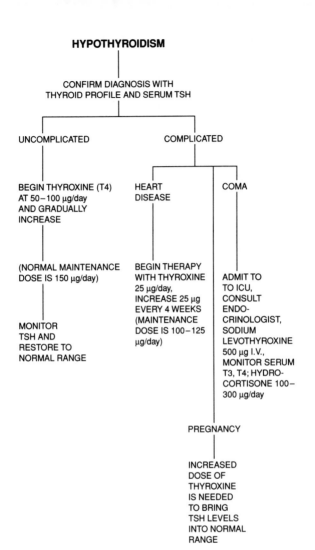

CONFIRM DIAGNOSIS WITH
THYROID PROFILE AND SERUM TSH

UNCOMPLICATED

COMPLICATED

BEGIN THYROXINE (T4)
AT 50–100 µg/day
AND GRADUALLY
INCREASE

HEART
DISEASE

COMA

(NORMAL MAINTENANCE
DOSE IS 150 µg/day)

MONITOR
TSH AND
RESTORE TO
NORMAL RANGE

BEGIN THERAPY
WITH THYROXINE
25 µg/day,
INCREASE 25 µg
EVERY 4 WEEKS
(MAINTENANCE
DOSE IS 100–125
µg/day)

ADMIT TO
TO ICU,
CONSULT
ENDO-
CRINOLOGIST,
SODIUM
LEVOTHYROXINE
500 µg I.V.,
MONITOR SERUM
T3, T4; HYDRO-
CORTISONE 100–
300 µg/day

PREGNANCY

INCREASED
DOSE OF
THYROXINE
IS NEEDED
TO BRING
TSH LEVELS
INTO NORMAL
RANGE

IDIOPATHIC POSTURAL HYPOTENSION

1. Confirm diagnosis by clinical picture.
2. Try antigravity stockings and increased salt intake first unless there are contraindications.
3. Next add fludrohydrocortisone 0.05−0.2 mg b.i.d.
4. Sympathomimetics and beta blockers may be tried.
5. Desmopressin or octreotide may also be tried in therapeutic doses. Consult an endocrinologist.

IDIOPATHIC PULMONARY FIBROSIS

1. Confirm diagnosis by chest x-ray, CT scans, pulmonary function testing, transbronchial or open lung biopsy. Consult a pulmonologist.
2. Oral corticosteroids such as prednisone 60–100 mg/day for 8–12 weeks, then gradually tapered to a maintenance level of 5–20 mg/day.
3. If the above treatment is not effective, add cyclophosphamide 1 mg/kg daily. Patient should continue the maintenance dose of prednisone.
4. Patient must stop smoking.
5. Supplemental oxygen may be necessary according to arterial blood gas analysis.
6. Treat right-sided heart failure with diuretics.
7. Patients should have flu and pneumococcal vaccines on appropriate schedule.
8. Consider lung transplant.

IMPETIGO

1. Confirm diagnosis by smear and culture of the lesions.
2. *Cases due to group A streptococci:*
   a. Oral penicillin V 500 mg q.i.d. p.o.
   b. Benzathine penicillin 300,000–1,200,000 units IM as a single dose if there is a question about compliance.
   c. Erythromycin 500 mg q.i.d. for patients who are allergic to penicillin.
3. *Cases due to Staphylococcus aureus:* Cefadroxil 30 mg/kg daily, given in divided doses q.12h. for children and 1 g/day for adults.
4. *Bullous impetigo occurring primarily in the newborn:* Dicloxacillin 25 mg/kg p.o. daily, divided into four doses.

IMPINGEMENT SYNDROME

1. Confirm diagnosis by MRI.
2. *Conservative treatment:*
   a. Avoid offending activity, nonsteroidal anti-inflammatory drugs.
   b. If the above is ineffective, try corticosteroid injection of subacromion bursa.
3. If conservative therapy fails, refer to an orthopedic surgeon for surgery.

INFECTIOUS MONONUCLEOSIS

1. Confirm diagnosis with blood smear, Monospot test, or heterophil antibody titer. Negative tests may warrant repeat titers.
2. Treatment is supportive, including bed rest and avoidance of contact sports; treat the fever with acetaminophen.
3. Corticosteroids may be necessary for complications such as airway obstruction, hemolytic anemia, or thrombocytopenia.
4. Chronic active EBV (Epstein–Barr virus) probably does not exist. It should not be included as a cause of chronic fatigue syndrome.

INFLUENZA

1. Confirm diagnosis by clinical evaluation and nose, throat, and sputum smears and cultures to rule out other pathogens.
2. *Uncomplicated cases:* Treat symptomatically. Avoid aspirin for patients under 18 years old.
3. Amantadine 200 mg/day may be given for influenza A viruses, especially in older patients or those with chronic lung disease.
4. Primary influenza pneumonia is treated with hospitalization and maintenance of oxygenation, hydration, and airway. Blood gases should be monitored frequently.
5. Observe for bacterial complications such as sinusitis and pneumonia.

Prophylaxis

Individuals with increased risk of complications from influenza should have vaccination. This includes patients with emphysema, cardiovascular disease, and immune deficiency and those over 65 years old. Amantadine may be administered for prophylaxis of influenza in high-risk groups.

INSULINOMA

1. Confirm diagnosis by taking frequent blood sugars during a 72-hour fast, plasma proinsulin, insulin, and C-peptide levels, and tolbutamide tolerance test. CT scan may help locate the tumor.
2. Maintain blood glucose levels with IV glucose infusion and octreotide administration.
3. Exploratory laparotomy and resection of tumor. If no tumor is found, a gradual pancreatectomy may be performed until a tumor is found on frozen section or until blood sugar rises to normal levels.
4. If there are metastases, the blood sugar can be controlled by octreotide or diazoxide. Consult an oncologist for chemotherapy.

INTRACRANIAL HEMORRHAGE

1. Confirm diagnosis with CT scans, initially, and MRI later. Avoid spinal tap.
2. *Control hypertension:*
   a. Mild: Sublingual nifedipine or oral propranolol.
   b. Moderate to severe: Labetalol.
3. *Control cerebral edema and increased intracranial pressure:* Treat with IV mannitol or other osmotic solutions.
4. *Maintain respiratory support:* Treat with intubation and mechanical ventilation.
5. *Cerebellar hemorrhage:*
   a. Greater than 3 cm: Surgical evacuation.
   b. Less than 3 cm. Observe.
6. *Cerebral hemorrhage:* Consider surgery, but this is controversial. Consult a neurosurgeon.
7. *Prognosis:* This is good for cerebellar hemorrhage but poor for cerebral and pontine hemorrhages.

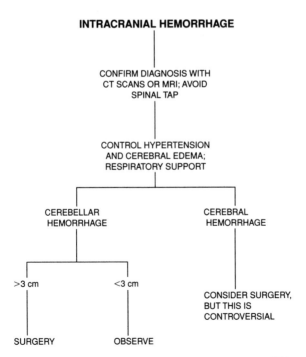

INTRACRANIAL HEMORRHAGE

CONFIRM DIAGNOSIS WITH CT SCANS OR MRI; AVOID SPINAL TAP

CONTROL HYPERTENSION AND CEREBRAL EDEMA; RESPIRATORY SUPPORT

CEREBELLAR HEMORRHAGE | CEREBRAL HEMORRHAGE

>3 cm | <3 cm

CONSIDER SURGERY, BUT THIS IS CONTROVERSIAL

SURGERY | OBSERVE

IRRITABLE BOWEL SYNDROME

1. Confirm diagnosis by history and exclusion of other causes of diarrhea, constipation, and abdominal pain.
2. High-fiber diet with supplements of psyllium (Metamucil, etc.) and bran.
3. Withdraw all laxatives.
4. Regular meals, regular exercise, and an attempt at defecation at a regular time each day.
5. For constipation, patient may use stool softeners (hemicellulose, etc.) or gentle low tap water enemas. Don't let this be overdone.
6. For diarrhea, patient may be prescribed diphenoxylate with atropine 10−20 mg q.i.d.
7. Psychotherapy when there is significant chronic anxiety or depression.
8. Antispasmodics may be helpful for cramps.

KALA-AZAR

1. Confirm diagnosis with bone marrow or lymph node aspiration and biopsy or splenic aspiration. Serologic tests may also be helpful.
2. Sodium antimony gluconate 20 mg/kg daily for 28 days. May have to repeat treatment with higher doses.
3. Alternatively, meglumine antimoniate or amphotericin B may be used. Consult an infectious disease specialist.
4. Pancytopenia may be treated with transfusions and splenectomy.
5. *Prevention:* This is best accomplished with elimination of diseased dogs and wiping out sandflies with DDT.

KLINEFELTER'S SYNDROME

1. Confirm diagnosis by buccal smear for sex chromatin, karyotype analysis, and serum FSH and LH. Testicular biopsy may also be helpful. Consult an endocrinologist.
2. Treat androgen deficiency with testosterone cypionate IM 200–400 mg monthly, but watch out for aggravation of gynecomastia.
3. Treat gynecomastia with surgery.
4. There is no treatment for the infertility.

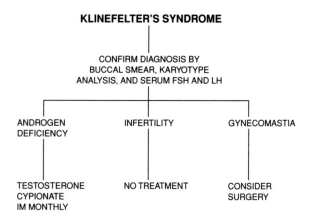

KORSAKOFF'S SYNDROME

1. Confirm diagnosis by history of alcoholism and blood alcohol levels.
2. Admit patient for alcohol withdrawal and rehabilitation.
3. Immediate administration of 100 mg of thiamine IV, followed by 50–100 mg/day orally or parenterally.
4. *Prognosis:* Only 25% of the patients achieve full recovery.

LACTASE DEFICIENCY

1. Confirm diagnosis by lactose tolerance test, hydrogen breath test, and measurement of lactase in a jejunal biopsy or lactase activity.
2. Treat with a lactose-free or lactose-restricted diet.

LANGERHANS' CELL GRANULOMATOSIS

1. Confirm diagnosis with lung or tissue biopsy.
2. *Unifocal:* Treat by excision or curettage. Rarely, radiation is necessary (consult a radiotherapist).
3. *Multifocal:* Consult an oncologist for treatment with methotrexate, prednisone, and vinblastine.

LARYNGITIS, ACUTE

1. Confirm diagnosis by laryngoscopy, smear and culture of exudates, lateral films of the neck to exclude epiglottitis, and clinical evaluation.
2. Children should be admitted to the intensive care unit to monitor for significant airway obstruction. Consult a pediatrician.
3. Adults may be treated at home with humidification, decongestants, and antibiotics when appropriate.
4. Corticosteroids have been recommended by some.

LEAD INTOXICATION

1. Confirm diagnosis by blood lead levels.
2. Remove patient from source of exposure.
3. Administer edetate calcium disodium (EDTA) intravenously up to 1.5 g per square meter of body surface area.
4. Alternatively, patient may receive penicillamine 20–40 mg/kg daily or dimercaprol up to 12–24 mg/kg daily.
5. May need combined edetate and dimercaprol therapy in acute encephalopathy.

LEGIONNAIRES' DISEASE

1. Confirm diagnosis by direct fluorescent antibody staining, cultures, and serologic tests.
2. Treat with erythromycin 500 mg q.6h. p.o. Lower doses must be used if there is renal or hepatic failure. Drug may be given IV up to 4 g/day in severe cases.
3. Alternative drugs are doxycycline or clarithromycin.
4. Add rifampin 600 mg b.i.d. in immunocompromised patients. Consult an infectious disease specialist.
5. *Prognosis:* Overall mortality is 15%.

LEISHMANIASIS, CUTANEOUS

1. Confirm diagnosis by smear and culture of aspirates or tissue or serologic tests. A skin test is also available.
2. Treat with sodium antimony gluconate intravenously 20 mg/kg daily for 20 days. May need to repeat.
3. Ketoconazole 600 mg/day for 28 days may be used for *Leishmania mexicana*.
4. An alternative drug is meglumine antimonate.

LEPROSY

1. Confirm diagnosis with smear of skin scrapings and with skin or nerve biopsies. Consult an infectious disease specialist or a leprologist.
2. Treat with dapsone 50–100 mg/day in a single dose. May add rifampin 600 mg/day.
3. Alternatively, clofazimine 50–200 mg/day may be given.
4. Combinations of the above drugs and older agents may be given under special circumstances.

LEPTOSPIROSIS

1. Confirm diagnosis with blood, urine, and spinal fluid cultures, guinea pig inoculation, and serologic tests.
2. Treat with IV penicillin G 1.5 million units q.6h. for 7 days. Doxycycline 100 mg b.i.d. may be more effective in jaundiced patients.
3. Watch for Jarisch–Herxheimer reaction.
4. *Prophylaxis:* Doxycycline 200 mg p.o. once a week may be used to prevent the disease.

LERICHE SYNDROME

1. Confirm diagnosis by aortography
2. Refer to cardiovascular surgeon for angioplasty, ondartoroctomy, or aortobifemoral bypass graft.

LEUKEMIA

1. Confirm diagnosis with CBC, blood smear, and bone marrow examination. Consult an oncologist for assistance in diagnosis and treatment.
2. *Acute myelogenous leukemia:* Treat with cytarabine, daunorubicin, or demethoxydaunorubicin. Consider bone marrow transplant. Monitor CBC.
3. *Acute lymphatic leukemia:* Treat with vincristine, prednisone, L-asparaginase, or daunorubicin. Consider bone marrow transplant. Monitor CBC.
4. *Chronic myelogenous leukemia:* Treatment may not be necessary. If it is, use busulphan 2–4 mg/24 hours orally. Monitor CBC.
5. *Chronic lymphatic leukemia:* Treatment is not always needed. Chlorambucil may be used to lower the lymphocyte count. If there is autoimmune hemolytic anemia, corticosteroids may be required. Radiotherapy may be useful for lymphadenopathy and splenomegaly. Monitor CBC.
6. Supportive care in the form of transfusions, prophylactic antibiotics and human immunoglobulin may be necessary.

LEUKEMIA

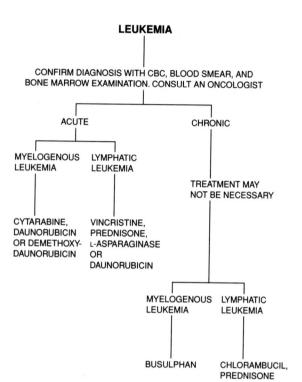

CONFIRM DIAGNOSIS WITH CBC, BLOOD SMEAR, AND
BONE MARROW EXAMINATION. CONSULT AN ONCOLOGIST

ACUTE

CHRONIC

MYELOGENOUS
LEUKEMIA

LYMPHATIC
LEUKEMIA

TREATMENT MAY
NOT BE NECESSARY

CYTARABINE,
DAUNORUBICIN
OR DEMETHOXY-
DAUNORUBICIN

VINCRISTINE,
PREDNISONE,
L-ASPARAGINASE
OR
DAUNORUBICIN

MYELOGENOUS
LEUKEMIA

LYMPHATIC
LEUKEMIA

BUSULPHAN

CHLORAMBUCIL,
PREDNISONE

LICHEN PLANUS

1. Confirm diagnosis with skin biopsy.
2. Treat with topical and systemic corticosteroids. Fluocinonide cream or ointment three times a day and prednisone 40–60 mg/day and gradually tapering is an acceptable combination.

LIPOPROTEINEMIAS

1. Confirm diagnosis by clinical findings, lipid profile, overnight plasma refrigeration, lipoprotein electrophoresis, and gel electrophoresis.
2. *Type I:* Fat-free diet and fat-soluble vitamins. Consult a dietician. Reduce calories also.
3. *Type II:* Low-fat diet. Transfusion of normal plasma may be helpful in severe cases. Consult a specialist in metabolic disease.
4. *Type III:* Look for and treat hypothyroidism. Control obesity and diabetes if present. If above measures are unsuccessful, give gemfibrozil or clofibrate.
5. *Familial hypercholsterolemia:* Low cholesterol, low saturated fat, high unsaturated fat diet. Administer cholestyramine, lovastatin, or nicotinic acid.
6. *Familial hypertriglyceridemia:* Caloric restriction, low saturated fat diet, gemfibrozil, nicotinic acid, and fish oil diet.
7. *Hypercholesterolemia unclassified:* Low cholesterol diet. If unsuccessful, lovastatin (Mevacor) or similar drugs.

Dosages

1. Gemfibrozil (Lopid) 0.6 g b.i.d.
2. Niacin 500–3000 mg/day.
3. Cholestyramine (Questran) 4–8 g one to two times a day.
4. Clofibrate (Atromid-S) 500 mg t.i.d. or q.i.d.
5. Lovastatin (Mevacor) 20–40 mg/day.
6. Simvastatin (Zocor), 5–20 mg/day.
7. Probucol (Lorelco) 1 gm/day.
8. Pravastatin sodium (Pravachol) 20–40 mg/day.

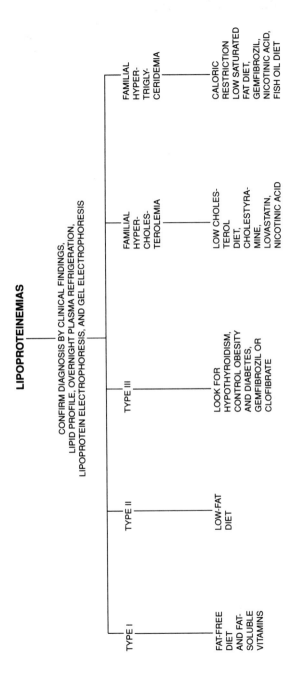

LIPOPROTEINEMIAS

CONFIRM DIAGNOSIS BY CLINICAL FINDINGS, LIPID PROFILE, OVERNIGHT PLASMA REFRIGERATION, LIPOPROTEIN ELECTROPHORESIS, AND GEL ELECTROPHORESIS

TYPE I

FAT-FREE DIET AND FAT-SOLUBLE VITAMINS

TYPE II

LOW-FAT DIET

TYPE III

LOOK FOR HYPOTHYROIDISM, CONTROL OBESITY AND DIABETES, GEMFIBROZIL OR CLOFIBRATE

FAMILIAL HYPER-CHOLES-TEROLEMIA

LOW CHOLES-TEROL DIET, CHOLESTYRA-MINE, LOVASTATIN, NICOTINIC ACID

FAMILIAL HYPER-TRIGLY-CERIDEMIA

CALORIC RESTRICTION LOW SATURATED FAT DIET, GEMFIBROZIL, NICOTINIC ACID, FISH OIL DIET

LISTERIOSIS

1. Confirm diagnosis by cultures of blood, spinal fluid, and amniotic fluid.
2. Treat with IV penicillin G 240,000–480,000 units/kg daily and gentamicin 6 mg/kg daily. Alternatively, IV ampicillin 150–300 mg/kg daily may be used with the gentamicin.
3. In penicillin-sensitive individuals, IV trimethoprim-sulfamethoxazole 15/75 mg/kg daily in three divided doses may be given.

LIVER ABSCESS

1. Confirm diagnosis by CT scans, ultrasonography, gallium or indium scans, serologic tests, or exploratory laparotomy.
2. Open or closed drainage. Consult an abdominal surgeon.
3. Treat with antibiotics or chemotherapy according to the results of cultures obtained from the abscess.

LIVER FAILURE

1. Confirm diagnosis by clinical assessment, liver function tests, EEG, and blood ammonia levels. Consult a gastroenterologist.
2. Admit to intensive care. Support vital signs.
3. Empty bowels with magnesium sulfate enemas, and restrict dietary protein.
4. Administer neomycin 1 g q.6h. to sterilize bowels.
5. Consider peritoneal or hemodialysis.
6. Avoid diuretics, sedatives, and other drugs.
7. Give cimetidine 200 mg q.8h. IV to keep gastric pH above 5.

LUNG ABSCESS

1. Confirm diagnosis by x-ray, bronchoscopy, CT scans, aspiration, and culture of exudate. Consult a pulmonologist.
2. Antibiotics are given for several weeks according to culture and sensitivity. Anaerobic cultures are necessary.
3. Postural drainage is helpful.
4. Surgical drainage is occasionally necessary.

LUPUS ERYTHEMATOSUS

1. Confirm diagnosis with ANA, L.E. preparation, antibodies to double-strand DNA (dsDNA), and biopsies. Consult a rheumatologist.
2. *Discoid lupus:* Treat with hydroxychloroquine 400 mg/day. Intralesional and systemic steroids may be used. Consult a dermatologist.
3. *Systemic lupus:*
   a. Mild: Treatment without the use of steroids can be successful. Myalgias, arthritis, fever, and serositis can be treated with NSAIDs. Reactions to these drugs are more common in this disease.
   b. Severe: Corticosteroids in large doses such as prednisone 1–2 mg/kg daily in two to three divided doses are indicated. These should be continued in large doses for 6–8 weeks and gradually tapered. A cytotoxic agent such as cyclophosphamide 1.5–2.5 mg/kg daily should be added if there is significant renal disease. It may be useful regardless.

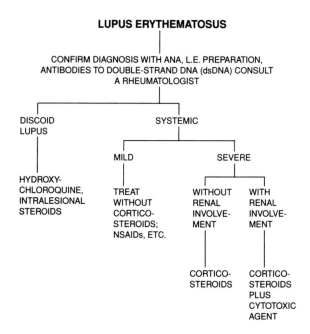

LYME DISEASE

1. Confirm diagnosis by serologic tests.
2. Treat adults (except during pregnancy) with doxycycline 100 mg b.i.d. for 10 days. Alternatively, amoxicillin 500 mg q.i.d. or cefuroxime 500 mg b.i.d. are effective. The latter two drugs may be given to pregnant women.
3. Children may be treated with amoxicillin 50 mg/kg daily or erythromycin 30 mg/kg daily.
4. For disseminated disease, the treatment should be administered for 20–30 days.
5. Some patients with arthritis may require synovectomy.
6. Patients with central nervous system disease need to receive their antibiotics intravenously—that is, ceftriaxone 2 g/day for 14–28 days. Consult a neurologist or an infectious disease specialist.

LYMPHANGITIS

1. Confirm diagnosis by history and physical examination.
2. Mild cases respond to procaine penicillin 600,000 units IM once or twice a day. Oral penicillin V 500–2000 mg/day may be used. Vancomycin 500–1000 mg IV q.12h. can be used if there is penicillin allergy or if *Staphylococcus* is suspected.
3. Severe cases are hospitalized and given large doses of penicillin IV (8–12 million units per day).
3. If the lymphangitis originated from a cat bite, amoxicillin-clavulanic acid 250–500 mg q.8h. may be used. For children, consult a pediatrician.

LYMPHOGRANULOMA VENEREUM

1. Confirm diagnosis with cultures, complement fixation test, and Frei test.
2. Treat with doxycycline 100 mg b.i.d. for 3 weeks.
3. Alternatively, erythromycin 500 mg q.i.d. may be used.

LYMPHOMA

1. Confirm diagnosis by x-rays, CT scans, biopsy, and staging laparotomy. Consult an oncologist for diagnosis and treatment.
2. *Hodgkin's lymphoma:*
   a. Stage IA, IIA, IB, IIB, and IIIA: Treat with radiotherapy alone or in combination with chemotherapy.
   b. Stage IIIB and IV: Treat with combination chemotherapy such as MOPP (mechlorethamine, vincristine, procarbazine, and prednisone). Alternatively, ABVD (Adriamycin, bleomycin, vinblastine, and dacarbazine) may be tried.
3. *Non-Hodgkin's lymphoma:*
   a. Stage I and II (low grade): Treat with radiotherapy. Radiotherapy and chemotherapy combined may occasionally be used.
   b. Stage III and IV: Treat with MOPP, CVP, or CHOP (cyclophosphamide, vincristine, doxorubicin, and prednisone). Consult an oncologist for numerous other treatment programs and bone marrow transplant.

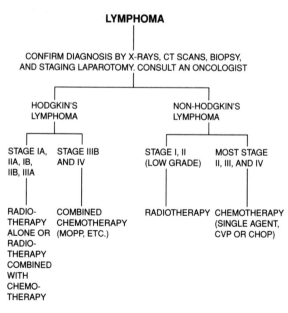

LYSOSOMAL STORAGE DISEASE

1. Confirm diagnosis by urinalysis, CBC, chemistry panel, x-rays, CT scans, and tissue biopsy.
2. Therapy is for the most part supportive. Consult a specialist in metabolic diseases. Genetic counseling is an important part of management.

MACROGLOBULINEMIA

1. Confirm diagnosis by CBC, blood smear, serum protein electrophoresis and immunoelectrophoresis, and tests for viscosity.
2. Hyperviscosity may be treated by plasmapheresis.
3. Treat with pulses of L-phenylalanine mustard, cyclophosphamide or chlorambucil, and prednisone 4–7 days every 4–6 weeks. Consult an oncologist.

MALABSORPTION SYNDROME

1. Confirm diagnosis with stool quantitative fat, D-xylose absorption test, bile acid breath test, and mucosal biopsy. Consult a gastroenterologist.
2. *Pancreatic insufficiency:* Treat with pancreatic enzymes.
3. *Celiac disease:* Treat with gluten-free diet. Consult a dietician.
4. *Tropical sprue:* Treat with vitamin B_{12}, folic acid, and doxycycline 100 mg b.i.d. for 14–28 days. Alternatively, a sulfonamide may be used.
5. *Whipple's disease:* Trimethoprim-sulfamethoxazole (160 mg and 800 mg, respectively) b.i.d. for 1 year.
6. *Intestinal lymphangiectasia:* Treat with a low-fat diet or substitute medium-chain triglycerides for long-chain triglycerides in the diet.

MALABSORPTION SYNDROME

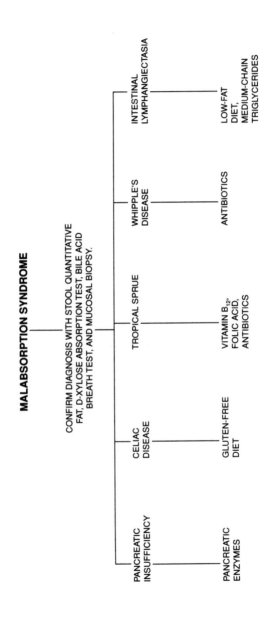

CONFIRM DIAGNOSIS WITH STOOL QUANTITATIVE FAT, D-XYLOSE ABSORPTION TEST, BILE ACID BREATH TEST, AND MUCOSAL BIOPSY.

PANCREATIC INSUFFICIENCY — PANCREATIC ENZYMES

CELIAC DISEASE — GLUTEN-FREE DIET

TROPICAL SPRUE — VITAMIN B_{12}, FOLIC ACID, ANTIBIOTICS

WHIPPLE'S DISEASE — ANTIBIOTICS

INTESTINAL LYMPHANGIECTASIA — LOW-FAT DIET, MEDIUM-CHAIN TRIGLYCERIDES

MALARIA

1. Confirm diagnosis with Giemsa stain of both thick and thin blood smears.
2. *Plasmodium falciparum:*
   a. If it is sensitive to chloroquine phosphate, this drug can be given orally in doses of 600 mg initially, followed by 300 mg 6, 24, and 48 hours later. Follow with blood smears.
   b. If it is resistant to chloroquine, give doxycycline 100 mg b.i.d. for 7 days with quinine sulfate 650 mg orally q.8h. for 3–7 days. In pregnant women and children under 8 years of age, use clindamycin 450 mg q.6h. for 3 days instead of doxycycline.
3. *Plasmodium vivax and ovale::* Treat with chloroquine phosphate as above, along with primaquine 15 mg/day for 2 weeks.
4. *Plasmodium malariae:* Treat with chloroquine alone according to schedule listed above.

Prophylaxis

Mefloquine 250 mg weekly for 4 weeks and then every week until leaving the endemic area. Alternatively, doxycycline 100 mg/day can be given until 4 weeks after leaving the endemic area. Mefloquine should be taken 1 week before entering the endemic area, and doxycycline should be taken 2 days before.

MALARIA

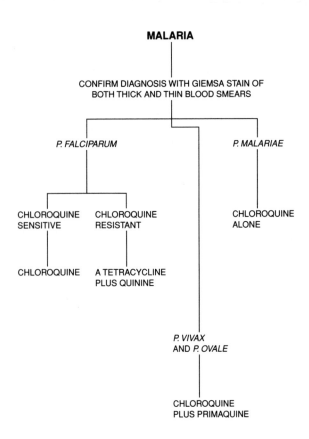

CONFIRM DIAGNOSIS WITH GIEMSA STAIN OF
BOTH THICK AND THIN BLOOD SMEARS

P. FALCIPARUM

P. MALARIAE

CHLOROQUINE
SENSITIVE

CHLOROQUINE
RESISTANT

CHLOROQUINE
ALONE

CHLOROQUINE

A TETRACYCLINE
PLUS QUININE

P. VIVAX
AND *P. OVALE*

CHLOROQUINE
PLUS PRIMAQUINE

MALLORY–WEISS TEAR

1. Confirm diagnosis by history and esophagoscopy. Consult a gastroenterologist.
2. Treatment is usually not necessary. Consult a gastroenterologist for endoscopic coagulation, intra-arterial vasopressin, or embolization.
3. Rarely, surgery may be required.

MARFAN'S SYNDROME

1. Confirm diagnosis with family history and physical, chest x-ray, slit-lamp examination, and the presence of homocystinuria.
2. No specific treatment is available, but beta blockers may delay aortic dilatation. Follow patients with echocardiography. Dislocated lens may occasionally require surgical treatment. Consult an ophthalmologist. Scoliosis is treated if greater than 20°. Consult an orthopedic surgeon.

MASTOIDITIS

1. Confirm diagnosis with x-rays of the mastoids. Consult an otolaryngologist.
2. Mild cases may be treated with trimethoprim-sulfamethoxazole (160 mg and 800 mg, respectively) twice daily in adults and half or less that dose in children (consult PDR for exact dose). Alternatively, amoxicillin-clavulanic acid (500 mg and 125 mg, respectively) t.i.d. may be used. Consult the PDR for dosages in children.
3. Moderate to severe cases should be referred immediately to an otolaryngologist for consideration for mastoidectomy.

McARDLE'S SYNDROME

1. Confirm diagnosis by muscle enzyme tests, myo-globinuria, and muscle biopsy. Consult a neurologist.
2. No specific treatment is available. Glucose or fructose before exercise may be helpful.

McCUNE–ALBRIGHT SYNDROME

1. Confirm diagnosis by clinical picture and x-rays of the skull and long bones.
2. No cure is available.
3. Calcitonin may be effective in the treatment of bone pain and high serum alkaline phosphatase.
4. Consult an orthopedic surgeon for casting, osteotomy, curettage, and so on.

MECKEL'S DIVERTICULUM

1. Diagnosis is usually not made until complications occur.
2. Confirm diagnosis of ulcer or ectopic gastric mucosa with isotope scan of abdomen after parenteral technetium. Consult an abdominal surgeon for treatment.
3. Confirm diagnosis of inflammation, obstruction, or rupture by exploratory laparotomy. Consult an abdominal surgeon.

MEDIASTINITIS

1. Confirm diagnosis by history of esophageal disease, instrumentation, or surgery. Consult a gastroenterologist and a thoracic surgeon for further diagnostic evaluation and treatment.
2. Treat with immediate surgical drainage and débridement and intravenous antibiotics.

MELANOMA

1. Confirm diagnosis by local excision biopsy. Consult a dermatologist.
2. Surgical excision is the treatment of choice. Palpable nodes should always be removed.
3. Chemotherapy is palliative in 25% of patients but rarely curative. Consult an oncologist.

MENIERE'S DISEASE

1. Confirm diagnosis by history, audiograms, nystagmography, and caloric testing. Consult a neurologist or an otolaryngologist.
2. Treatment of the acute attacks is symptomatic. Meclizine 12.5–25 mg is effective in reducing the vertigo. If there is vomiting, prochlorperazine 12.5 mg is administered intramuscularly.
3. Patients should refrain from alcohol and cigarettes. Bioflavonoids 1–2 capsules three times a day has been effective in reducing the number of attacks in this author's experience. Betahistine 8 mg q.8h. may also reduce the frequency and severity of attacks. A high-potassium, low-sodium diet has been advocated by some.
4. If the attacks become disabling, a shunting procedure or surgical destruction of the labyrinth may be necessary. Consult an otolaryngologist.

MENINGITIS

1. Confirm diagnosis by spinal fluid analysis, smear, and culture. A CT scan of the brain should be done first if there is papilledema or focal neurologic signs. Consult a neurologist.
2. *Viral meningitis:* Hospitalize the patient, apply isolation procedures and obtain viral studies. Observe the patient for the development of encephalitis.
3. *Bacterial meningitis:* Hospitalize in isolation (in the intensive care unit if the patient is critically ill). Until the diagnosis is established, begin IV penicillin G 2 million units q.2h. and IV ceftriaxone 2 g q.12h. Consult a pediatrician for guidance in treating children.
   a. *Neisseria meningitidis:* Treat with IV penicillin G 2 million units q.2h until patient is afebrile for 5 days. If penicillin-sensitive, treat with ceftriaxone or chloramphenicol.
   b. *Hemophilus influenza:* Treat with IV ceftriaxone 2 g q.12h. for 10–14 days. If penicillin-sensitive, use chloramphenicol.
   c. *Streptococcus pneumoniae:* Treat with IV penicillin G 2 million units q.2h. for 10–14 days. If patient is sensitive to penicillin, treat with chloramphenicol IV 1.0–1.5 g q.6h. or vancomycin.
   d. Listeria monocytogenes: See page 260.

Prophylaxis

This is important for patients exposed to *N. meningitidis.* In these patients, give rifampin 600 mg q.12h. for 2 days.

MENINGITIS

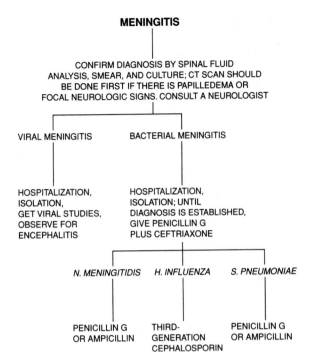

CONFIRM DIAGNOSIS BY SPINAL FLUID
ANALYSIS, SMEAR, AND CULTURE; CT SCAN SHOULD
BE DONE FIRST IF THERE IS PAPILLEDEMA OR
FOCAL NEUROLOGIC SIGNS. CONSULT A NEUROLOGIST

VIRAL MENINGITIS

BACTERIAL MENINGITIS

HOSPITALIZATION,
ISOLATION,
GET VIRAL STUDIES,
OBSERVE FOR
ENCEPHALITIS

HOSPITALIZATION,
ISOLATION; UNTIL
DIAGNOSIS IS ESTABLISHED,
GIVE PENICILLIN G
PLUS CEFTRIAXONE

N. MENINGITIDIS

H. INFLUENZA

S. PNEUMONIAE

PENICILLIN G
OR AMPICILLIN

THIRD-
GENERATION
CEPHALOSPORIN

PENICILLIN G
OR AMPICILLIN

MENINGOCOCCEMIA

1. Confirm diagnosis with clinical findings and blood, spinal fluid, synovial fluid, or petechial scrapings for smear and culture. Serologic tests may also be done.
2. Treat with IV penicillin G 2 million units q.2h. If the patient is sensitive to penicillin, chloramphenicol may be used. The pediatric dose of penicillin is 200,000–300,000 units per kilogram of body weight. This is given IV q.4h. Consult a pediatrician.

MENOPAUSE

1. Confirm diagnosis by history and physical, Pap smear, and serum FSH and estradiol. When in doubt, consult a gynecologist.
2. *Patients without a contraindication for estrogen therapy:*
   a. With a hysterectomy: Treat with estrogen therapy alone, such as ethinyl estradiol 0.01–0.02 mg/day for 25 days per month.
   b. Without a hysterectomy: Treat with estrogen plus progesterone, such as ethinyl estradiol 0.01–0.02 mg/day for 25 days per month and medroxyprogesterone 10 mg/day the last 10–13 days of estrogen administration. A new combined estrogen and progesterone preparation (Prempro) may be used alternatively for 21–25 days per month.
3. *Patients with a contraindication for estrogen therapy (such as carcinoma of the breast or uterus):*
   a. With hot flashes: These respond to 50–150 mg of medroxyprogesterone every 3 months. Clonidine may also be helpful.
   b. Osteoporosis: Calcium 1000–1500 mg/day, such as two calcium carbonate tablets (e.g., Tums) three to four times a day. Etidronate 400 mg/day for 2 weeks every 3 months. Alendronate sodium (Fosamax) tablets may be given at a dose of 10 mg a day. Consult a gynecologist for guidance. Calcitonin and fluoride may also be used.

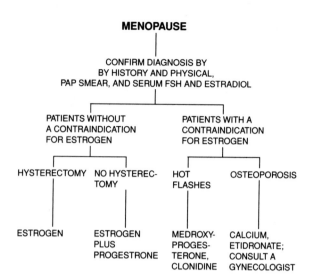

MENOPAUSE

CONFIRM DIAGNOSIS BY
BY HISTORY AND PHYSICAL,
PAP SMEAR, AND SERUM FSH AND ESTRADIOL

PATIENTS WITHOUT
A CONTRAINDICATION
FOR ESTROGEN

PATIENTS WITH A
CONTRAINDICATION
FOR ESTROGEN

HYSTERECTOMY

NO HYSTEREC-
TOMY

HOT
FLASHES

OSTEOPOROSIS

ESTROGEN

ESTROGEN
PLUS
PROGESTRONE

MEDROXY-
PROGES-
TERONE,
CLONIDINE

CALCIUM,
ETIDRONATE;
CONSULT A
GYNECOLOGIST

MESENTERIC ARTERY INSUFFICIENCY, EMBOLISM, OR THROMBOSIS

1. Confirm diagnosis by history and physical and mesenteric angiography. Consult a cardiovascular surgeon.
2. *Insufficiency:* Treat with balloon angioplasty, stent, or bypass grafts.
3. *Embolism:* Treat with embolectomy or bowel resection.
4. *Thrombosis:* Treat with bowel resection.

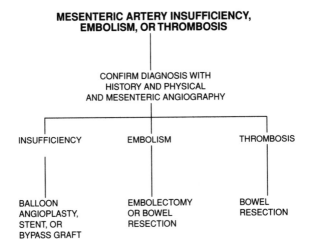

METHEMOGLOBINEMIA AND SULFHEMOGLOBINEMIA

1. Confirm diagnosis by history of exposure to drugs or toxins and no change in the color of blood on exposure to air. The absorbance of sulfhemoglobin is not decreased by the addition of cyanide, but the absorbance of methemoglobin is.
2. Treat toxic methemoglobinemia with methylene blue 2 mg/kg IV over a 1-hour period. This may be repeated if necessary. Consult a hematologist.

MIGRAINE

1. Confirm diagnosis by history and superficial temporal artery compression during attack. Observe response to sublingual ergotamine or oral or subcutaneous sumatriptan.
2. *Treatment of attack:*
   a. Give sumatriptan 25–100 mg orally or 3–6 mg subcutaneously.
   b. If poor response, try prochlorperazine 5–10 mg IV and/or diphenhydramine 50–100 mg IV slowly. Consult a neurologist before trying narcotics.
   c. If poor response, admit for IV fluids, oxygen, corticosteroids, and narcotics.
3. *Prophylaxis:*
   a. Tyramine-free diet for all patients.
   b. In children use cyproheptadine 2–4 mg q.i.d. or phenytoin 50–300 mg/day. Consult a neurologist.
   c. In adults with menstrual migraine, use a combination of ergotamine and a nonsteroidal anti-inflammatory agent (naproxen 500 mg b.i.d.). Medroxyprogesterone 150 mg IM every 3–4 months may be used to suppress menstruation. Consult a gynecologist.
   d. In most adults, use a long-acting beta blocker such as atenolol 25–100 mg/day or metoprolol 50–200 mg/day. Propranolol may be tried. When beta blockers are ineffective alone, a tricyclic antidepressant such as nortriptyline 10–50 mg at bedtime may be tried alone or in combination with a beta blocker. Consult a neurologist for assistance in using other prophylactic drugs such as anticonvulsants, calcium channel blockers, and serotonin antagonists.

MIGRAINE

CONFIRM DIAGNOSIS BY
HISTORY AND SUPERFICIAL TEMPORAL
ARTERY COMPRESSION DURING AN ATTACK,
RESPONSE TO ERGOTAMINE

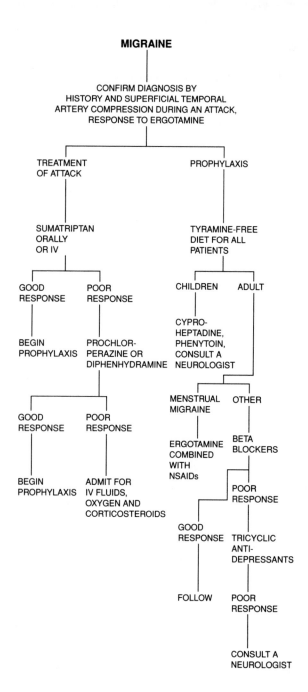

TREATMENT
OF ATTACK

PROPHYLAXIS

SUMATRIPTAN
ORALLY
OR IV

TYRAMINE-FREE
DIET FOR ALL
PATIENTS

GOOD
RESPONSE

POOR
RESPONSE

CHILDREN   ADULT

BEGIN
PROPHYLAXIS

PROCHLOR-
PERAZINE OR
DIPHENHYDRAMINE

CYPRO-
HEPTADINE,
PHENYTOIN,
CONSULT A
NEUROLOGIST

GOOD
RESPONSE

POOR
RESPONSE

MENSTRUAL
MIGRAINE

OTHER

BEGIN
PROPHYLAXIS

ADMIT FOR
IV FLUIDS,
OXYGEN AND
CORTICOSTEROIDS

ERGOTAMINE
COMBINED
WITH
NSAIDs

BETA
BLOCKERS

POOR
RESPONSE

GOOD
RESPONSE

TRICYCLIC
ANTI-
DEPRESSANTS

FOLLOW

POOR
RESPONSE

CONSULT A
NEUROLOGIST

MILROY'S DISEASE

1. Confirm diagnosis by family history and exclusion of other causes of lymphoma.
2. Treat with frequent elevation of lower limbs, exercise, graduated compression hose, and skin care. Intermittent pneumatic compression devices may be indicated. Consult an expert in peripheral vascular disease.

MITRAL VALVULAR DISEASE

1. Confirm diagnosis by history, physical examination, EKG, chest x-ray, and echocardiography. Consult a cardiologist.
2. *Mitral valve prolapse:*
   a. Asymptomatic: Treat with reassurance and prophylactic antibiotics during surgery and dental procedures.
   b. Arrhythmias: Consult a cardiologist.
   c. Atypical chest pain: Beta blockers, consult a cardiologist.
   d. Embolism: Consult a cardiologist for use of antiplatelet drugs and Coumadin.
3. *Mitral stenosis:*
   a. Asymptomatic: Reassurance and antibiotic prophylaxis for streptococcal infections and for surgical and dental procedures.
   b. Symptomatic patients: Consult a cardiologist or cardiovascular surgeon for evaluation for valvulotomy.
   c. Atrial fibrillation: Consult a cardiologist. If it is acute or relatively recent, try cardioversion (medically or electrically). If it is chronic long-standing, surgery should be considered. Anticoagulants should be considered in patients who are a poor surgical risk. Look for coexisting hyperthyroidism.
4. *Mitral regurgitation:*
   a. Asymptomatic: Reassurance and prophylactic antibiotics for prevention of streptococcal infections and before and during surgical and dental procedures.
   b. Mildly symptomatic: Salt restriction, diuretics, ACE inhibitors, and restriction of physical activities. Consult a cardiologist for guidance.
   c. Moderate to severe: Consider surgery. Consult a cardiologist.

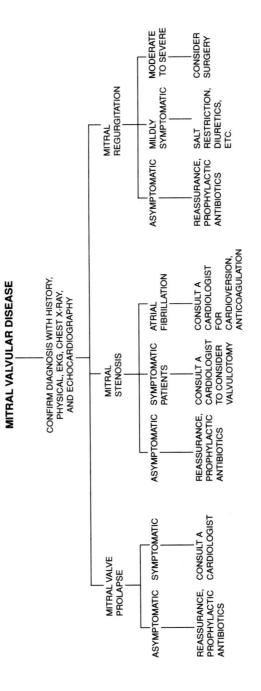

MITRAL VALVULAR DISEASE

CONFIRM DIAGNOSIS WITH HISTORY, PHYSICAL, EKG, CHEST X-RAY, AND ECHOCARDIOGRAPHY

MITRAL VALVE PROLAPSE

- ASYMPTOMATIC → REASSURANCE, PROPHYLACTIC ANTIBIOTICS
- SYMPTOMATIC → CONSULT A CARDIOLOGIST

MITRAL STENOSIS

- ASYMPTOMATIC → REASSURANCE, PROPHYLACTIC ANTIBIOTICS
- SYMPTOMATIC PATIENTS → CONSULT A CARDIOLOGIST TO CONSIDER VALVULOTOMY
- ATRIAL FIBRILLATION → CONSULT A CARDIOLOGIST FOR CARDIOVERSION, ANTICOAGULATION

MITRAL REGURGITATION

- ASYMPTOMATIC → REASSURANCE, PROPHYLACTIC ANTIBIOTICS
- MILDLY SYMPTOMATIC → SALT RESTRICTION, DIURETICS, ETC.
- MODERATE TO SEVERE → CONSIDER SURGERY

MUCORMYCOSIS

1. Confirm diagnosis with wet smear of crushed tissue, sputum smear and culture, and tissue biopsy. Consult an infectious disease specialist.
1. Amphotericin B IV for 10−12 weeks (page 33).
3. Regulate coexisting diabetes mellitus.
4. Consult a surgeon for débridement of craniofacial lesions.
5. *Prognosis:* Fifty percent of patients with infections limited to the head and face can survive. Survival is rare in infections elsewhere.

MULTIPLE MYELOMA

1. Confirm diagnosis by serum protein electrophoresis and immunoelectrophoresis, bone marrow examination, and urine for Bence Jones protein.
2. Treat active cases with an alkylating agent such as melphalan, cyclophosphamide (or chlorambucil), and prednisone. Consult an oncologist for guidance. Polychemotherapy seems to have a higher rate of initial response. However, long-term survival doesn't seem to have improved.
3. Supportive care includes irradiation and analgesics for bone pain, steroids for hypercalcemia, and plasmapheresis for hyperviscosity syndromes. Consult an oncologist.

MULTIPLE SCLEROSIS

1. Confirm the diagnosis by MRIs of the brain and spinal cord, evoked potential studies, and spinal fluid analysis for gamma globulin and myelin basic protein.
2. *Acute attack:* Treat with methylprednisolone 20 mg q.i.d. p.o. or 1 g/day IV for 5−7 days and then gradually taper. ACTH may be useful (see page 30).
3. *Chronic relapsing form:* Give 45 million units of beta interferon subcutaneously every other day to decrease the frequency and severity of attacks. Avonex TM (interferon beta-1a) may also be used by weekly IM injections.
4. Supportive care includes a low-fat diet, multiple vitamins, regular exercise, and weekly vitamin B_{12} injections or daily vitamin B_{12} by mouth.
5. Patients should avoid high altitudes, crowded rooms, vaccination, excessive heat and cold, stress, and exhaustive exercise.
6. Physical therapy for advanced forms of the disease with spasticity, and so on.
7. Baclofen 10−20 mg q.i.d. for spasticity.

MUMPS

1. Confirm diagnosis with serologic tests, viral isolation, and skin test.
2. There is no specific treatment. Supportive care includes regular mouth care, analgesics, and a bland diet.
3. Corticosteroids may be of value in reducing testicular pain and swelling. Treat with prednisone 1 mg/kg daily initially for 7–10 days and then gradually taper.
4. *Prevention:* Mumps vaccine is administered to children after reaching 1 year of age and to adults who have never had clinical mumps or the vaccine.

MUSCULAR DYSTROPHY

1. Confirm diagnosis by family history, electromyography, and muscle biopsy.
2. Treatment is for the most part supportive. Prednisone 0.75 mg/kg daily may decrease the progression for 1–3 years in Duchenne muscular dystrophy.
3. The myotonia in various forms of muscular dystrophy can be treated with anticonvulsants such as phenytoin.

MYASTHENIA GRAVIS

1. Confirm diagnosis with blood anti-acetylcholine receptor antibody, edrophonium response test, and electromyography. Look for a thymoma. Consult a neurologist.
2. Consider thymectomy for all patients between puberty and 55 years of age.
3. *Mild myasthenia:* Treat first with anticholinesterase drugs such as pyridostigmine 60 mg 3–5 times daily. Use the edrophonium response test to evaluate the need for increasing the dose. May gradually introduce corticosteroids.
4. *Chronic mild to moderate myasthenia:* Treat first with corticosteroids such as prednisone 15–25 mg/day and gradually increase until there is substantial clinical improvement or a maximum of 50 mg/day has been reached. That dose is continued for 1–3 months and then transferred to an alternate-day schedule. The dose is then gradually reduced until the minimum dose needed to maintain control is reached. The drug is then continued indefinitely.
5. Other immunosuppressants may be used (e.g., cyclophosphamide, azathioprine, etc.). Consult an oncologist for guidance.
6. *Myasthenic crisis:* Admit the patient to the intensive care unit and insert endotracheal tube. Consult an anesthesiologist. All anticholinesterase drugs are stopped and then gradually restarted with frequent evaluations with edrophonium. Plasmapheresis should be considered. Consult a neurologist. If it is desirable to introduce corticosteroids, these can be given in large doses immediately while the patient is intubated.

MYASTHENIA GRAVIS

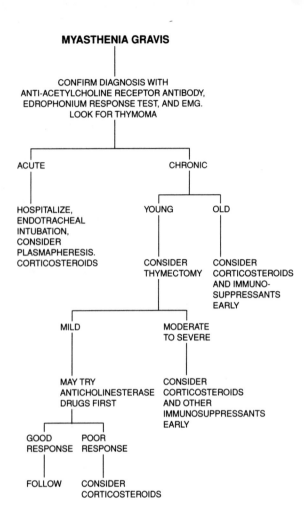

CONFIRM DIAGNOSIS WITH
ANTI-ACETYLCHOLINE RECEPTOR ANTIBODY,
EDROPHONIUM RESPONSE TEST, AND EMG.
LOOK FOR THYMOMA

ACUTE

CHRONIC

HOSPITALIZE,
ENDOTRACHEAL
INTUBATION,
CONSIDER
PLASMAPHERESIS.
CORTICOSTEROIDS

YOUNG

OLD

CONSIDER
THYMECTOMY

CONSIDER
CORTICOSTEROIDS
AND IMMUNO-
SUPPRESSANTS
EARLY

MILD

MODERATE
TO SEVERE

MAY TRY
ANTICHOLINESTERASE
DRUGS FIRST

CONSIDER
CORTICOSTEROIDS
AND OTHER
IMMUNOSUPPRESSANTS
EARLY

GOOD
RESPONSE

POOR
RESPONSE

FOLLOW

CONSIDER
CORTICOSTEROIDS

MYOCARDIAL INFARCTION

1. Confirm diagnosis by serial EKGs, serial cardiac enzymes, and imaging studies. Consult a cardiologist.
2. Admit to coronary care unit.
3. *Uncomplicated:*
   a. If admitted within 6 hours of onset (the exact time is debatable), consider thrombolytic therapy or percutaneous transluminal coronary angioplasty (PTCA).
   b. If not admitted within 6 hours of onset, treat with aspirin, oxygen, oral or intravenous nitroglycerin, narcotics, and beta blockers. Ask a cardiologist for guidance.
4. *Complicated:*
   a. Congestive heart failure without shock: May treat initially with furosemide 40–80 mg IV and nitroglycerin. If not improved, a Swan–Ganz catheter is passed and treatment is based on the pulmonary capillary wedge pressure. If it is greater than 18 mm, continue diuretics and nitroglycerin. If it is less than 18 mm, then IV fluids should be pushed.
   b. Arrhythmias: See Cardiac Arrhythmias, page 61.
   c. Shock: Enlist the help of a cardiologist. First insert a Swan–Ganz catheter to determine the pulmonary capillary wedge pressure. If it is low, administer IV fluids, especially normal saline. Consider PTCA or thrombolytic therapy if patient is seen early. If the hypotension is not caused by hypovolemia, administer vasopressors such as dopamine and Dobutrex. Aortic counterpulsation may be helpful. If IV fluids and vasopressors fail to alleviate the situation, consider a ruptured ventricular septum or papillary muscle, myocardial rupture and tamponade, and so on.

MYOCARDIAL INFARCTION

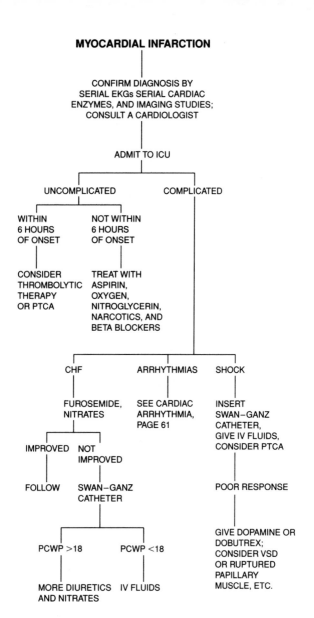

CONFIRM DIAGNOSIS BY
SERIAL EKGs SERIAL CARDIAC
ENZYMES, AND IMAGING STUDIES;
CONSULT A CARDIOLOGIST

ADMIT TO ICU

UNCOMPLICATED   COMPLICATED

WITHIN   NOT WITHIN
6 HOURS   6 HOURS
OF ONSET   OF ONSET

CONSIDER   TREAT WITH
THROMBOLYTIC   ASPIRIN,
THERAPY   OXYGEN,
OR PTCA   NITROGLYCERIN,
                NARCOTICS, AND
                BETA BLOCKERS

CHF   ARRHYTHMIAS   SHOCK

FUROSEMIDE,   SEE CARDIAC   INSERT
NITRATES   ARRHYTHMIA,   SWAN–GANZ
                PAGE 61   CATHETER,
                                GIVE IV FLUIDS,
                                CONSIDER PTCA

IMPROVED NOT   POOR RESPONSE
          IMPROVED

FOLLOW   SWAN–GANZ   GIVE DOPAMINE OR
          CATHETER   DOBUTREX;
                                CONSIDER VSD
                                OR RUPTURED
PCWP >18   PCWP <18   PAPILLARY
                                MUSCLE, ETC.

MORE DIURETICS IV FLUIDS
AND NITRATES

MYOTONIA ATROPHICA

1. Confirm diagnosis with family history, electromyography, and muscle biopsy.
2. No specific therapy available. Myotonia may be treated with anticonvulsant drugs such as phenytoin 200–400 mg/day.

NARCOLEPSY

1. Confirm diagnosis by history and wake and sleep EEG.
2. Treat initially with pemoline 18.75 mg, up to 6 tablets per day. If this is unsuccessful, methylphenidate 5–10 mg t.i.d. may be used. Amphetamines may also be effective.
3. Cataplectic attacks may be reduced by imipramine 25 mg t.i.d.

NEPHROLITHIASIS

1. Confirm diagnosis by 24-hour urines, chemistry panel, parathyroid hormone studies, urine oxalate, citrate and cystine, intravenous pyelogram, diagnostic ultrasonography and stone analysis.
2. *Acute attack:* Hospitalize for sedation and parenteral narcotic analgesics. Consult a urologist for treatment with extracorporeal or percutaneous lithotripsy or fragmentation of the stone by endoscopic passage of an ultrasonic transducer into the ureter via cystoscopy.
3. *Prophylaxis:*
   a. Calcium stones: Increase fluid intake to 6−8 glasses a day; prescribe hydrochlorothiazide 50 mg/day. Potassium citrate may be added also.
   b. Uric acid stones: Treat with supplemental sodium bicarbonate 1−3 mmol/kg daily. Add 250 mg of acetazolamide twice daily. Use allopurinol 300 mg/day.
   c. Struvite stones: Treat with daily administration of methenamine mandelate. In some cases, NH_4Cl may be used, but this may promote the formation of oxalate stones.
   d. Cystine stones: Treat with hydration to keep urine volume at 3 liters/day. Use sodium bicarbonate to raise urine pH. Consult a urologist for additional techniques.

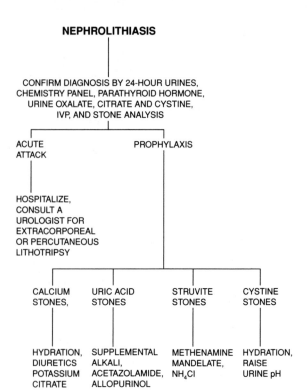

NEPHROLITHIASIS

CONFIRM DIAGNOSIS BY 24-HOUR URINES,
CHEMISTRY PANEL, PARATHYROID HORMONE,
URINE OXALATE, CITRATE AND CYSTINE,
IVP, AND STONE ANALYSIS

ACUTE
ATTACK

PROPHYLAXIS

HOSPITALIZE,
CONSULT A
UROLOGIST FOR
EXTRACORPOREAL
OR PERCUTANEOUS
LITHOTRIPSY

CALCIUM
STONES,

URIC ACID
STONES

STRUVITE
STONES

CYSTINE
STONES

HYDRATION,
DIURETICS
POTASSIUM
CITRATE

SUPPLEMENTAL
ALKALI,
ACETAZOLAMIDE,
ALLOPURINOL

METHENAMINE
MANDELATE,
NH_4Cl

HYDRATION,
RAISE
URINE pH

NEPHROTIC SYNDROME, IDIOPATHIC

1. Confirm diagnosis with renal biopsy. Consult a nephrologist.
2. Treat all patients with general measures such as high-protein, high-caloric diet, fluid restriction, and diuretics. Don't overdo diuretics. A thiazide diuretic may be tried first, but loop diuretics are usually needed.
3. *Minimal-change disease:* Corticosteroids are usually successful in reducing the albuminuria and edema. Prednisone 1.0–1.5 mg/kg daily is given for 4 weeks and then tapered to alternate-day schedule. Tapering must be gradual as relapses occur if tapering is too abrupt. If there are frequent relapses, another immunosuppressant such as cyclophosphamide 2–3 mg/kg daily may be tried.
4. *Focal glomerulosclerosis:* Corticosteroids may be tried, although they are successful in only 20–40%. Other immunosuppressants may be tried.
5. *Membranous glomerulonephritis:* Treat with alternate-day corticosteroids such as 125 mg of prednisone every other day for several weeks and judiciously taper. A combination of corticosteroids and other immunosuppressant drugs may be effective.
6. *Membranoproliferative glomerulonephritis:* Treatment with corticosteroids may delay the progression of the disease, but the use of steroids with other immunosuppressants has not proved beneficial. Long-term alternate-day prednisone 20–30 mg every other day (or 0.3–0.5 mg/kg every other day) is utilized. Anticoagulants and platelet aggregation inhibitors may be useful.

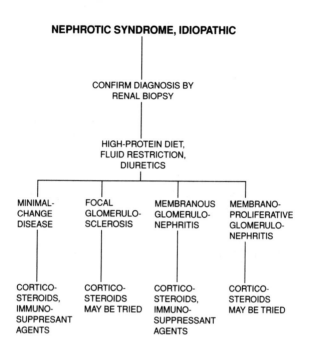

NEPHROTIC SYNDROME, IDIOPATHIC

CONFIRM DIAGNOSIS BY
RENAL BIOPSY

HIGH-PROTEIN DIET,
FLUID RESTRICTION,
DIURETICS

| MINIMAL-CHANGE DISEASE | FOCAL GLOMERULO-SCLEROSIS | MEMBRANOUS GLOMERULO-NEPHRITIS | MEMBRANO-PROLIFERATIVE GLOMERULO-NEPHRITIS |

CORTICO-STEROIDS, IMMUNO-SUPPRESSANT AGENTS

CORTICO-STEROIDS MAY BE TRIED

CORTICO-STEROIDS, IMMUNO-SUPPRESSANT AGENTS

CORTICO-STEROIDS MAY BE TRIED

NEUROBLASTOMA

1. Confirm diagnosis by CT scan of the abdomen, intravenous pyelography, ultrasonography, urinary catecholamine, and bone marrow examination. Consult an oncologist.
2. Treat with surgical excision, followed by radiation or chemotherapy. Consult an oncologist.

NEUROFIBROMATOSIS

1. Confirm diagnosis by family history, physical examination, and biopsy.
2. Treat with surgical excision of the tumors when they cause functional difficulties (i.e., acoustic neuromas, page 4) or cosmetic problems.

NEUROMA, TRAUMATIC

1. Confirm diagnosis by history, physical, and exploration and biopsy.
2. Treat by excision and, when functionally necessary, reanastomosis of the nerve endings.

NIEMANN–PICK DISEASE

1. Confirm by history, physical examination, bone marrow examination, and enzyme assay.
2. No specific treatment is available.

NOCARDIOSIS

1. Confirm diagnosis with acid-fast smears, culture, bronchoscopy, needle aspiration, and lung biopsy.
2. Treat with sulfisoxazole 6–8 g/day, divided into four doses. Doses up to 12 g/day may be necessary.
3. Alternatively, minocycline 100–200 mg b.i.d. may be utilized.
4. In resistant cases, choice of drug should be based on culture and sensitivity studies. Consult an infectious disease specialist.

NUTRITIONAL ANEMIA

1. Confirm diagnosis by CBC, blood smear for red cell morphology, serum iron, iron binding capacity and ferritin, serum vitamin B_{12} and folic acid, and bone marrow examination in difficult cases.
2. *Iron-deficiency anemia:* Give ferrous sulfate 300 mg one to three times daily as tolerated. If the patient is unable to tolerate iron tablets or capsules, try liquid iron. If the patient is still unable to tolerate iron orally, administer intravenous iron dextran with the dose calculated by the following formula:

$$\text{mg of iron} = 0.3 \times \text{body wt. in lbs.} \times \left(100 - \frac{\text{hemoglobin} \times 100}{14.8}\right)$$

   It is preferable to give the iron IV slowly after a test dose of 1–2 drops.
3. *Vitamin B_{12} deficiency:* Vitamin B_{12} 1000 μg IM is given three times weekly for 4–6 weeks, and then 1000 μg is administered monthly for life.
4. *Folic acid deficiency:* Vitamin B_{12} 1000 μg/day is administered for 3 days and then folic acid 1 mg/day is given until CBC is normal. Maintenance dose depends on the clinical diagnosis. If there is a malabsorption syndrome, the folic acid must be given parenterally.
5. Observe reticulocyte response after each form of therapy to confirm that working diagnosis was correct.

NUTRITIONAL ANEMIA

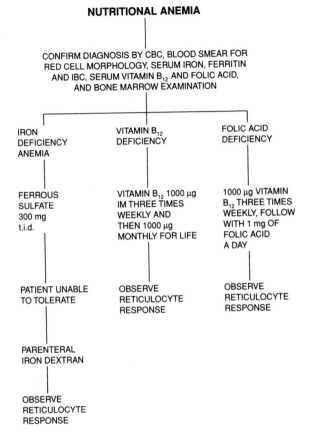

CONFIRM DIAGNOSIS BY CBC, BLOOD SMEAR FOR
RED CELL MORPHOLOGY, SERUM IRON, FERRITIN
AND IBC, SERUM VITAMIN B_{12} AND FOLIC ACID,
AND BONE MARROW EXAMINATION

IRON
DEFICIENCY
ANEMIA

FERROUS
SULFATE
300 mg
t.i.d.

PATIENT UNABLE
TO TOLERATE

PARENTERAL
IRON DEXTRAN

OBSERVE
RETICULOCYTE
RESPONSE

VITAMIN B_{12}
DEFICIENCY

VITAMIN B_{12} 1000 μg
IM THREE TIMES
WEEKLY AND
THEN 1000 μg
MONTHLY FOR LIFE

OBSERVE
RETICULOCYTE
RESPONSE

FOLIC ACID
DEFICIENCY

1000 μg VITAMIN
B_{12} THREE TIMES
WEEKLY, FOLLOW
WITH 1 mg OF
FOLIC ACID
A DAY

OBSERVE
RETICULOCYTE
RESPONSE

OBESITY

1. Confirm diagnosis by history, physical examination, and excluding secondary causes such as hypothyroidism, Cushing's disease, and insulinoma.
2. Treat initially with low-calorie balanced diet, regular exercise, group therapy or psychotherapy, and weekly visits to the doctor's office.
3. If the above program is unsuccessful, a diet consisting of fruits and vegetables in unlimited amounts, four slices of whole wheat bread per day, and fish, chicken, or turkey twice per week may be tried. Patients generally need an appetite suppressant such as phentermine HCl 30 mg q.d. to assist in cooperating with diet. The patient should be allowed to go off the diet one day a week to ensure compliance.
4. Appetite suppression may be enhanced by the combination of phentermine HCl 30 mg/day and fenfluramine HCl 20 mg t.i.d. Dexfenfluramine HCL (Redux TM) 15 mg b.i.d. is also effective.
5. Surgery may be necessary if the patient is massively overweight, conventional measures have failed, and the obesity is life-threatening. Gastric bypass and gastroplasty seem to be the best procedures. Referral to a center that specializes in these procedures is recommended.

Alternative Appetite Suppressants

1. Diethylpropion HCl 25 mg t.i.d. or 75 mg of a timed-release tablet once a day.
2. Phenmetrazine HCl 25 mg t.i.d. or a 50- to 75-mg timed-release tablet once a day.
3. Mazindol 1–2 mg/day.

OPTIC NEURITIS

1. Confirm diagnosis by history, physical, visual field examination, and visual evoked potential study. Consult an ophthalmologist.
2. Treat acute cases with IV methylprednisolone 1000 mg/day for 3 days, followed by oral methylprednisolone 16−28 mg/day and gradually tapering over a 3-week period.

ORCHITIS

1. Confirm diagnosis by history, physical examination, and careful exclusion of torsion of the testicle. Do urethral smear and culture after prostatic massage.
2. If the orchitis is secondary to prostatitis or epididymitis from gonorrhea or other bacteria, treat with appropriate antibiotics (page 138).
3. If the orchitis is due to mumps, treat with prednisone 40 mg/day for 4 days and gradually taper.

OROYA FEVER

1. Confirm diagnosis by CBC, red cell fragility tests, chromium tagged red cell survival times, and blood cultures.
2. Treat with chloramphenicol 50–100 mg/kg daily in four to six divided doses. Alternatively, tetracycline and penicillin may be used. Consult an infectious disease specialist.

OSTEOARTHRITIS

1. Confirm diagnosis by physical examination, x-rays, and exclusion of other forms of arthritis.
2. If there is obesity, weight reduction is important. Exercise is important to all patients.
3. *Primarily large joint involvement:* Treat with nonsteroidal anti-inflammatory agents first. If unsuccessful, intra-articular corticosteroids may be used, such as triamcinolone diacetate 20–40 mg in 3–4 cc of 1% lidocaine. These should not be given frequently because of the risk of damage to the cartilage. If there is no improvement, consult an orthopedic surgeon for arthroscopy and/or evaluation for joint replacement.
4. *Primarily small joint involvement:* Treat with nonsteroidal anti-inflammatory agents and physical therapy. Intra-articular joint injections may be utilized in selected cases. Consult a rheumatologist.

Dosages

1. Ibuprofen (Motrin): 400–800 mg t.i.d.
2. Naproxen (Naprosyn): 250–500 mg t.i.d.
3. Piroxicam (Feldene): 20 mg q.d.
4. Sulindac (Clinoril): 150–200 mg b.i.d.
5. Indomethacin (Indocin): 25–50 mg q.i.d.
6. Prednisone 30–60 mg q.d. and gradually taper over 10- to 20-day period.
7. *Intra-articular steroids:*
   a. Triamcinolone diacetate 20–40 mg/cc.
   b. Betamethasone sodium phosphate and acetate suspension (Celestone Soluspan) 6 mg/cc.

OSTEOARTHRITIS

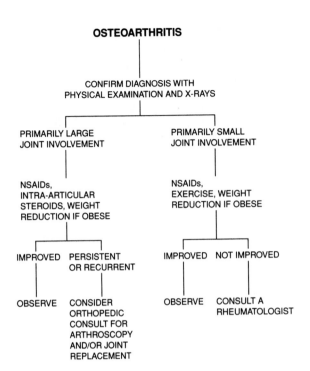

CONFIRM DIAGNOSIS WITH
PHYSICAL EXAMINATION AND X-RAYS

PRIMARILY LARGE
JOINT INVOLVEMENT

PRIMARILY SMALL
JOINT INVOLVEMENT

NSAIDs,
INTRA-ARTICULAR
STEROIDS, WEIGHT
REDUCTION IF OBESE

NSAIDs,
EXERCISE, WEIGHT
REDUCTION IF OBESE

IMPROVED   PERSISTENT
OR RECURRENT

IMPROVED   NOT IMPROVED

OBSERVE   CONSIDER
ORTHOPEDIC
CONSULT FOR
ARTHROSCOPY
AND/OR JOINT
REPLACEMENT

OBSERVE   CONSULT A
RHEUMATOLOGIST

OSTEOGENESIS IMPERFECTA

1. Confirm diagnosis by history, physical examination, and x-rays.
2. No specific treatment has been found.
3. Supportive measures such as exercise, physical therapy, counseling, and treatment of the fractures are indicated. Consult an orthopedic surgeon and physiatrist.

OSTEOGENIC SARCOMA

1. Confirm diagnosis by x-rays, bone scans, and alkaline phosphatase levels.
2. Treat by augmentation and wide resection, chemotherapy, or radiation. Consult an oncologist and a radiotherapist.
3. *Prognosis:* Poor because pulmonary metastases are often present at the time of resection.

OSTEOMALACIA

1. Confirm diagnosis with serum calcium, phosphorus, and alkaline phosphatase and with x-rays of the bones.
2. Treat with vitamin D_2 or D_3 800–4000 units daily for 8–12 weeks, followed by maintenance dosages. Be sure and administer adequate calcium supplements concomitantly.

OSTEOMYELITIS

1. Confirm diagnosis by x-rays, bone scans, and MRI. Obtain cultures of exudates before beginning antibiotic therapy, if possible. Consult an orthopedic surgeon.
2. Antibiotic therapy is based on the results of cultures unless the condition is critical. In that case, therapy is started before cultures are completed. Empirical therapy should include a drug that is active against *Staphylococcus aureus,* such as oxacillin or a cephalosporin and an aminoglycoside to combat gram-negative organisms. Antibiotics must be continued for weeks in the acute cases and sometimes for months in chronic cases.
3. Surgery is often not necessary in acute osteomyelitis, but it is usually indicated in chronic osteomyelitis.

OSTEOPETROSIS

1. Confirm diagnosis by x-rays of skull and long bones.
2. *Mild cases:* Symptomatic treatment of fractures, and so on.
3. *Severe cases:* Bone marrow transplants and calcitriol therapy. Consult an orthopedic surgeon.

OSTEOPOROSIS

1. Confirm diagnosis by plain x-rays of bone, dual energy x-ray absorptiometry, and quantitative computed tomography.
2. Estrogens are administered to postmenopausal women (see page 287).
3. Testosterone preparations are given to men with gonadal deficiency; 200–400 mg of testosterone propionate in oil once a month should be adequate.
4. Calcium 1500 mg is administered daily in divided doses. Low doses of vitamin D (800 units/day) are also useful.
5. For women who cannot take estrogen, etidronate or alendronate sodium (Fosamax) tablets 10 mg daily is given.
6. Calcitonin may also be used. Consult an endocrinologist. It can be given in doses of 50 units subcutaneously every other day or 200 units/day by nasal spray.

Dosages of Various Oral Calcium Preparations

1. Oscal 500–1250 mg calcium carbonate from oyster shell and 500 mg elemental calcium each tablet.
2. Tums–500 mg calcium carbonate and 200 mg elemental calcium each tablet.

OSTEOPOROSIS

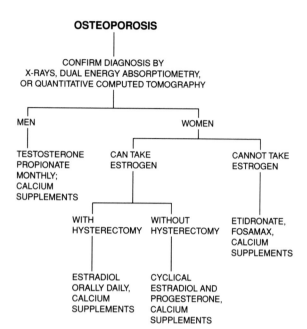

CONFIRM DIAGNOSIS BY
X-RAYS, DUAL ENERGY ABSORPTIOMETRY,
OR QUANTITATIVE COMPUTED TOMOGRAPHY

MEN

TESTOSTERONE
PROPIONATE
MONTHLY;
CALCIUM
SUPPLEMENTS

WOMEN

CAN TAKE
ESTROGEN

WITH
HYSTERECTOMY

ESTRADIOL
ORALLY DAILY,
CALCIUM
SUPPLEMENTS

WITHOUT
HYSTERECTOMY

CYCLICAL
ESTRADIOL AND
PROGESTERONE,
CALCIUM
SUPPLEMENTS

CANNOT TAKE
ESTROGEN

ETIDRONATE,
FOSAMAX,
CALCIUM
SUPPLEMENTS

OTITIS EXTERNA

1. Confirm diagnosis by history, physical examination, and cultures.
2. Gentle irrigation with hypertonic saline or a solution of two-thirds rubbing alcohol and one-third vinegar will remove debris.
3. Topical polymyxin B/neomycin drops four times a day will be sufficient for mild infections.
4. Moderate to severe infections require systemic antibiotics such as dicloxacillin 500 mg q.i.d. or cephalexin 500 mg q.i.d. Consult an otolaryngologist, especially if incision and drainage is considered necessary.

OTITIS MEDIA

1. Confirm diagnosis by history, physical examination, and culture of transtympanic aspirate if necessary.
2. Treat with systemic antibiotics such as trimethoprim 160 mg and sulfamethoxazole 800 mg b.i.d. or amoxicillin-clavulanate 250–500 mg t.i.d. for 7–10 days.
3. Alternatively, a cephalosporin may be used.
4. Treat pain with local anesthetic solution (Auralgan, etc.) or systemic analgesics.
5. Consult an otolaryngologist for evaluation for myringotomy.
6. If condition becomes chronic, consult an otolaryngologist.

OVARIAN CANCER

1. Confirm diagnosis with serum CA 125 determination, transvaginal ultrasonography, and exploratory laparotomy.
2. Consult a gynecologist for bilateral salpingo-oophorectomy, total abdominal hysterectomy, and staging.
3. Consult an oncologist for evaluation for chemotherapy in advanced-stage disease and adjuvant therapy following surgery in stage I and II cancers.

PAGET'S DISEASE

1. Confirm diagnosis by skeletal survey (x-rays), bone scans, and marked elevation of the plasma alkaline phosphatase.
2. No treatment necessary in the majority of cases.
3. Treat pain with NSAIDs such as indomethacin 25 mg q.i.d.
4. Calcitonin 50–100 NRC units subcutaneously may reduce pain, slow the progression of the disease, and improve neurologic symptomatology. Consult an endocrinologist.
5. Etidronate and Fosamax reduces bone resorption. Consult an endocrinologist for guidance.

PANCREATITIS

1. Confirm diagnosis with serum and urinary amylase, serum lipase, CT scans, and ultrasonography.
2. *Acute:*
   a. Hospitalize for nasogastric suction, IV fluids, and analgesics such as meperidine 50–100 mg q.4h. IM or IV and atropine gr 1/150.
   b. If patient fails to respond, consider pancreatic pseudocyst, abscess, hypocalcemia, and diabetes. Consult a gastroenterologist and a surgeon.
   c. Transfusions and plasma expanders may be necessary if shock develops.
3. *Chronic:* Avoid alcohol, administer pancreatic enzymes if there is evidence of malabsorption, and treat diabetes and other complications. Consult a gastroenterologist. May need large doses of pancreatic enzymes or surgery for relief of pain.

PANCREATITIS

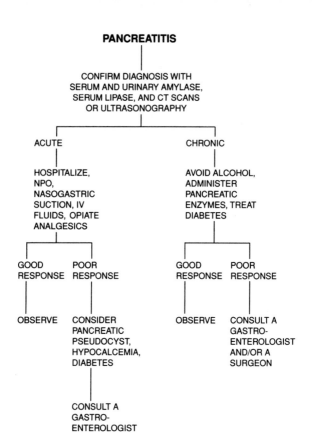

CONFIRM DIAGNOSIS WITH
SERUM AND URINARY AMYLASE,
SERUM LIPASE, AND CT SCANS
OR ULTRASONOGRAPHY

ACUTE

CHRONIC

HOSPITALIZE,
NPO,
NASOGASTRIC
SUCTION, IV
FLUIDS, OPIATE
ANALGESICS

AVOID ALCOHOL,
ADMINISTER
PANCREATIC
ENZYMES, TREAT
DIABETES

GOOD
RESPONSE

POOR
RESPONSE

GOOD
RESPONSE

POOR
RESPONSE

OBSERVE

CONSIDER
PANCREATIC
PSEUDOCYST,
HYPOCALCEMIA,
DIABETES

OBSERVE

CONSULT A
GASTRO-
ENTEROLOGIST
AND/OR A
SURGEON

CONSULT A
GASTRO-
ENTEROLOGIST

PANNICULITIS, ACUTE

1. Confirm diagnosis by tissue biopsy.
2. Search for the cause.
3. Treat with combined chemotherapy such as cyclophosphamide, bleomycin, and prednisone. Consult an oncologist for guidance. Results of treatment are generally poor.

PARALYSIS AGITANS

1. Confirm diagnosis by neurologic examination. Exclude drug and manganese toxicity.
2. For all cases, prescribe exercise, physical therapy, or psychotherapy.
3. Mild or early cases:
   a. Try a course of amantadine 100 mg b.i.d.
   b. If treatment a is ineffective, try deprenyl 5 mg b.i.d.
   c. If treatment b is ineffective, the treatment is the same as for advanced forms of the disease.
4. Moderate to severe:
   a. Treat with 1:4 ratio of carbidopa and levodopa (such as 25–100 mg t.i.d.) initially. May need to gradually increase dose to 200 mg carbidopa and 2000 mg levodopa to get adequate response.
   b. If the patient becomes refractory to the above therapy or has a poor response, add a dopamine receptor agonist such as bromocriptine or pergolide. Consult a neurologist for guidance.
   c. If the patient is young and becomes refractory to the above therapy, refer to a neurosurgeon for adrenal medullary transplants or stereotactic surgery.

PARALYSIS AGITANS

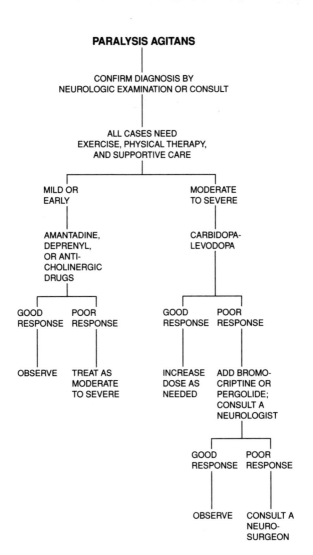

CONFIRM DIAGNOSIS BY
NEUROLOGIC EXAMINATION OR CONSULT

ALL CASES NEED
EXERCISE, PHYSICAL THERAPY,
AND SUPPORTIVE CARE

MILD OR EARLY

AMANTADINE, DEPRENYL, OR ANTI-CHOLINERGIC DRUGS

GOOD RESPONSE — OBSERVE

POOR RESPONSE — TREAT AS MODERATE TO SEVERE

MODERATE TO SEVERE

CARBIDOPA-LEVODOPA

GOOD RESPONSE — INCREASE DOSE AS NEEDED

POOR RESPONSE — ADD BROMO-CRIPTINE OR PERGOLIDE; CONSULT A NEUROLOGIST

GOOD RESPONSE — OBSERVE

POOR RESPONSE — CONSULT A NEURO-SURGEON

Paralysis Agitans 339

PELLAGRA

1. Confirm diagnosis by history, physical examination, and response to niacin.
2. Treat with niacin 10−50 mg t.i.d. and high-protein diet.
3. Patient should also receive adequate doses of other vitamins.

PEMPHIGUS VULGARIS

1. Confirm diagnosis by skin biopsy. Consult a dermatologist.
2. Treat first with corticosteroids such as prednisone 1.0–1.5 mg/kg daily.
3. If corticosteroids alone are inadequate, immediately add an immunosuppressant agent such as cyclophosphamide 1 mg/kg daily. Consult a dermatologist for guidance.

PEPTIC ULCER

1. Acute complicated by severe hemorrhage or perforation: Consult a surgeon.
2. *Acute uncomplicated or chronic:* Confirm diagnosis by endoscopy and biopsy with urease testing or serologic tests for *H. pylori.*
3. *Tests positive for H. pylori:*
   a. Treat with omeprazole 20 mg b.i.d., and clarithromycin 500 mg t.i.d. or amoxicillin 500 mg q.i.d. for 2 weeks and continue omeprazole for an additional 2 weeks.
   b. Alternatively, use omeprazole 20 mg b.i.d., clarithromycin 500 mg b.i.d., and metronidazole 500 mg b.i.d. for 2 weeks, and continue omeprazole for 4 weeks altogether.
   c. Be sure and begin omeprazole simultaneously with antibiotics.
4. *Tests negative for H. pylori:*
   a. Uncomplicated: Treat with H2-receptor antagonist such as ranitidine HCl 150 mg b.i.d.
   b. Complicated (history of perforation or bleeding): Treat with omeprazole and clarithromycin according to the above schedule.
   c. Poor response to omeprazole and clarithromycin: Treat with other antibiotics or H2-receptor antagonist.
   d. Fails to respond to above measures: Consult an abdominal surgeon.

PEPTIC ULCER

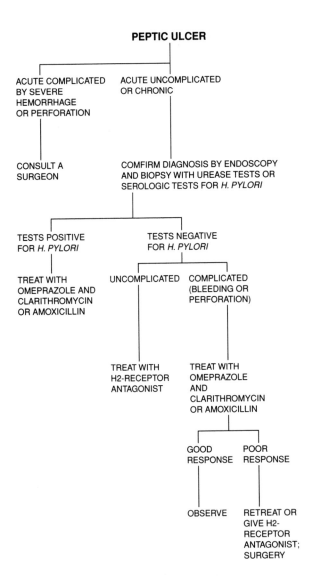

PERIARTERITIS NODOSA

1. Confirm diagnosis by biopsy of the involved tissues (renal, etc.) or angiography of involved arteries.
2. Treat with prednisone 1 mg/kg daily and cyclophosphamide 1 mg/kg daily for 6–12 weeks and gradually taper. Consult an oncologist.
3. Treat complications such as hypertension, renal failure, and so on. Consult a rheumatologist.

PERICARDITIS

1. Confirm diagnosis by chest x-rays, EKG, and echocardiography or CT scans. Consult a cardiologist. Look for cause.
2. *Acute:*
   a. Hospitalize and observe for pericardial effusion or tamponade.
   b. No effusion: Treat pain with NSAIDs such as aspirin 650 mg q.4h. If poor response, try prednisone 1 mg/kg daily for 1 week and gradually taper.
   c. Effusion: Consult a cardiologist for pericardiocentesis.
3. *Chronic:*
   a. Effusion: Pericardiocentesis. If no improvement, consider pericardial resection.
   b. No effusion: Consider pericardial resection.

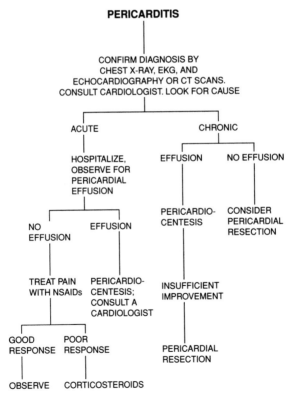

PERINEPHRIC ABSCESS

1. Confirm diagnosis with ultrasonography and/or CT scans.
2. Consult a urologist for percutaneous drainage of abscess.
3. Administer antibiotics based on cultures of the exudate. Consult an infectious disease specialist in resistant cases.

PERIPHERAL NEUROPATHY

1. Confirm diagnosis with electrodiagnostic studies and electromyography. Consider neurology consult early.
2. Confirm types of neuropathy with spinal fluid analysis, glucose tolerance testing, urine prophyrins, blood lead level, urine arsenic, and so on.
3. *Guillain–Barré syndrome:* Hospitalize, respiratory support, plasma exchange, immunoglobulin infusion, corticosteroids, neurology consult.
4. *Heavy metal neuropathy:* Chelation therapy, neurology consult.
5. *Porphyria:* Glucose infusion, IV hemin, neurology consult.
6. *Diabetic neuropathy:* Control blood sugar, improve nutrition, add high-dose vitamin B; use tricyclics and anticonvulsants or topical capsaicin for pain.
7. *Uremic neuropathy:* Hemodialysis, renal transplant, consult a nephrologist.
8. *Inherited neuropathy:* No treatment available.
9. *Chronic demyelinating inflammatory neuropathy:* Corticosteroids, immunosuppressants, neurology consult (see page 183).
10. *Toxic neuropathy:* Withdraw drug or toxin.

Dosages

1. *Plasma exchange:* 3.0–3.5 liters per day every other day for 6–10 days.
2. *Corticosteroids:* Prednisone 60–100 mg/day for 8–12 weeks and gradually taper.
3. *Chelation therapy:*
   a. BAL 2.5 mg/kg q.i.d. for 2 days, b.i.d. for another day, and then once daily for 10 days.
   b. D-Penicillamine 250 mg q.i.d. and continue until urine arsenic falls below 25 μg in 24 hours.
4. *Glucose infusions:* 500 g per 24 hours.
5. *Hemin IV:* 1–4 mg/kg daily for up to 14 days.

6. *Tricyclics:*
   a. Amitriptyline 10–150 mg/day.
   b. Trazadone 50–200 mg/day.
7. *Anticonvulsants:*
   a. Phenytoin 300–600 mg/day.
   b. Carbamazepine 600–1200 mg/day.
8. *Topical capsaicin:* 0.025–0.075% cream 2–3 times daily.

PERIPHERAL NEUROPATHY

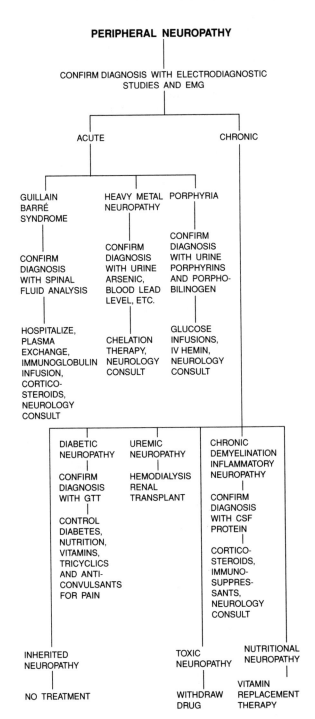

CONFIRM DIAGNOSIS WITH ELECTRODIAGNOSTIC STUDIES AND EMG

ACUTE

CHRONIC

GUILLAIN BARRÉ SYNDROME

CONFIRM DIAGNOSIS WITH SPINAL FLUID ANALYSIS

HOSPITALIZE, PLASMA EXCHANGE, IMMUNOGLOBULIN INFUSION, CORTICO-STEROIDS, NEUROLOGY CONSULT

HEAVY METAL NEUROPATHY

CONFIRM DIAGNOSIS WITH URINE ARSENIC, BLOOD LEAD LEVEL, ETC.

CHELATION THERAPY, NEUROLOGY CONSULT

PORPHYRIA

CONFIRM DIAGNOSIS WITH URINE PORPHYRINS AND PORPHO-BILINOGEN

GLUCOSE INFUSIONS, IV HEMIN, NEUROLOGY CONSULT

DIABETIC NEUROPATHY

CONFIRM DIAGNOSIS WITH GTT

CONTROL DIABETES, NUTRITION, VITAMINS, TRICYCLICS AND ANTI-CONVULSANTS FOR PAIN

UREMIC NEUROPATHY

HEMODIALYSIS RENAL TRANSPLANT

CHRONIC DEMYELINATION INFLAMMATORY NEUROPATHY

CONFIRM DIAGNOSIS WITH CSF PROTEIN

CORTICO-STEROIDS, IMMUNO-SUPPRES-SANTS, NEUROLOGY CONSULT

INHERITED NEUROPATHY

NO TREATMENT

TOXIC NEUROPATHY

WITHDRAW DRUG

NUTRITIONAL NEUROPATHY

VITAMIN REPLACEMENT THERAPY

PERITONITIS

1. Confirm diagnosis by history and physical, para-centesis and cultures of peritoneal fluid and blood. Consult a surgeon.
2. *Primary peritonitis:* Treat with a cephalosporin such as cefotaxime until culture and sensitivity studies are available.
3. *Secondary peritonitis:*
   a. Begin cefotetan 2 g q.12h. IV and metronida-zole with a loading dose of 15 mg/kg, fol-lowed by 7.5 mg/kg q.6h. IV.
   b. Ampicillin may be used alternatively.
   c. Prepare for surgery.
   d. Change antibiotics according to culture and sensitivity studies.

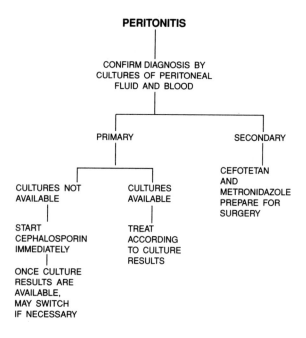

PERNICIOUS ANEMIA

1. Confirm diagnosis with CBC, blood smear, serum vitamin B_{12} and folic acid, Schilling test, and bone marrow examination.
2. Treat with 1000 µg of vitamin B_{12} IM three times weekly for 4–6 weeks and then 1000 µg of vitamin B_{12} IM monthly. Follow with CBC and reticulocyte counts in early stages.

PERONEAL MUSCULAR ATROPHY

1. Confirm diagnosis with family history, nerve conduction velocity studies, EMG, and nerve biopsy. Consult a neurologist.
2. No specific treatment available.
3. Orthopedic appliances such as foot drop braces are useful. Consult an orthopedic surgeon.

PERONEAL NEUROPATHY

1. Confirm diagnosis by nerve conduction velocity studies and electromyography. Consult a neurologist. Rule out systemic causes (diabetes, etc.).
2. Treat with therapeutic doses of vitamin B complex, physiotherapy, and foot drop braces.

PERTUSSIS

1. Confirm diagnosis by nasopharyngeal swab cultures and serological tests.
2. Treat with erythromycin 50 mg/kg daily in four divided doses for 14 days.
3. Alternatively, trimethoprim/sulfamethoxazole 8/40 mg/kg daily is given in two divided doses.
4. *Prevention:*
    a. Treat all contacts irrespective of immunization status as above.
    b. Pertussis vaccine is given as DTP beginning at 6–8 weeks of age in three doses with 2-month intervals. Booster doses are given at 15–18 months and four to 6 years of age.

PEUTZ-JEGHERS SYNDROME

1. Confirm diagnosis by clinical examination, family history, upper GI series, barium enema, and endoscopic studies.
2. Treat with surgical removal of the polyps as indicated.

PEYRONIE'S DISEASE

1. Confirm diagnosis with clinical evaluation and urological consult.
2. Treat with excision of plaque and skin graft and other procedures as proposed by a urologist. Medical treatment is of little proven value.

PHARYNGITIS AND TONSILLITIS

1. Confirm diagnosis by smear and culture, rapid strept tests, and serologic tests.
2. *Streptococcal pharyngitis:*
   a. Children under 12: Treat with penicillin V 250 mg t.i.d. for 10 days.
   b. All other patients: Penicillin V 500 mg t.i.d. for 10 days.
   c. Use parenteral penicillin (benzathine penicillin G 600,000–900,000 units) only on patients who cannot be relied upon to take the medication. Be sure they are not allergic to penicillin.
   d. Alternatively, erythromycin 20–40 mg/kg daily is given.
3. *Gonococcal pharyngitis:* Treat with ceftriaxone 250 mg IM, followed by doxycycline 100 mg b.i.d. for 7 days.

PHARYNGOCONJUNCTIVAL FEVER

1. Confirm diagnosis by cultures and serologic tests.
2. No specific treatment is available.

PHENYLPYRUVIC OLIGOPHRENIA

1. Confirm diagnosis by family history, clinical picture, urine PKU tests, and plasma phenylalanine. Consult a pediatrician.
2. Treat with a diet that replaces protein with an amino acid mixture low in phenylalanine. Consult a dietician. Maintain plasma phenylalanine between 180 and 700 μmol/liter (3–12 mg/dl).

PHEOCHROMOCYTOMA

1. Confirm diagnosis by 24-hour urine VMA, metanephrines, or fractionated unconjugated ("free") catecholamines. CT scans of abdomen and chest and aortography are used to locate the site of the tumor.
2. Treat with surgical removal of the tumor after preoperative alpha-adrenergic blockade. Phenoxybenzamine in doses of 40–200 mg is given for 10–14 days before surgery. Consult an endocrinologist.
3. Unresectable or malignant tumors: Consult an oncologist.
4. *Prognosis:* Recurrence rate is only 10%. Follow patient with frequent assessment of 24-hour urine catecholamines.

PHLEBOTOMUS FEVER

1. Confirm diagnosis by history, physical examination, and geographic location.
2. Treatment is symptomatic.

PINEALOMA

1. Confirm diagnosis with CT scans and MRIs of the brain.
2. Treat with surgery, radiation, and chemotherapy. Consult a neurosurgeon and an oncologist.
3. *Prognosis:* These tumors have a 60–80% 5-year survival with radiation.

PINWORM DISEASE

1. Confirm the diagnosis by applying clear cellulose acetate tape to the anus in the morning and transferring the tape to a microscope slide for examination.
2. Treat with mebendazole 100 mg as a single dose and repeat in 14 days. Treat all members of the family or household.

PITUITARY ADENOMA

1. Confirm diagnosis by CT scans, MRIs, and assays of blood and urine pituitary and target organ hormones (prolactin, growth hormone, ACTH, cortisol, etc.). Consult an endocrinologist.
2. *Patients who are good operative risks:*
   a. Microadenomas and tumors confined to the sella turcica: Treat with transsphenoidal hypophysectomy.
   b. Large tumors and those with suprasellar extension: Either transsphenoidal or subfrontal approach can be used, and both may be used together. Radiotherapy should follow surgery.
3. *Patients who are a poor operative risk:*
   a. With small tumors with no visual or endocrinological deficit, observation may be best.
   b. Small tumors with endocrine hypersecretion may be treated with radiation.
   c. Large tumors with visual deterioration require surgery, followed by radiation if there is incomplete removal.

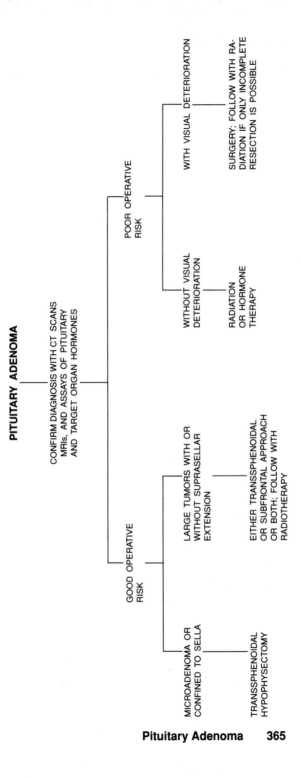

PITUITARY ADENOMA

CONFIRM DIAGNOSIS WITH CT SCANS MRIs, AND ASSAYS OF PITUITARY AND TARGET ORGAN HORMONES

GOOD OPERATIVE RISK

MICROADENOMA OR CONFINED TO SELLA

TRANSSPHENOIDAL HYPOPHYSECTOMY

LARGE TUMORS WITH OR WITHOUT SUPRASELLAR EXTENSION

EITHER TRANSSPHENOIDAL OR SUBFRONTAL APPROACH OR BOTH; FOLLOW WITH RADIOTHERAPY

POOR OPERATIVE RISK

WITHOUT VISUAL DETERIORATION

RADIATION OR HORMONE THERAPY

WITH VISUAL DETERIORATION

SURGERY; FOLLOW WITH RA-DIATION IF ONLY INCOMPLETE RESECTION IS POSSIBLE

Pituitary Adenoma   365

PITYRIASIS ROSEA

1. Confirm diagnosis by clinical examination and skin biopsy.
2. No specific treatment is necessary because the eruption resolves spontaneously over a 2- to 6-week period.
3. Treat pruritus with hydroxyzine orally or topical steroids.

PLAGUE

1. Confirm diagnosis by culture of aspiration material from buboes or sputum, blood cultures, and serologic tests. Consult an infectious disease specialist.
2. Treat with streptomycin 7.5–15 mg/kg q.12h. for 10 days.
3. Alternatively, tetracycline and chloramphenicol may be used. Chloramphenicol is the drug of choice in meningitis or hypotensive patients.

PNEUMOCONIOSIS

1. Confirm diagnosis by history of exposure to coal dust, silica, or asbestos, along with chest x-ray and pulmonary function tests. Open lung biopsy is rarely indicated.
2. No specific therapy is available, but removal from exposure is indicated as soon as the diagnosis is established.
3. Treat pulmonary fibrosis, emphysema, and right heart failure symptomatically. See discussion of treatment under their respective headings. Observe patients with asbestos exposure for mesentheliomas.

PNEUMOCYSTIS CARINII

1. Confirm diagnosis by sputum staining with special reagents (toluidine blue, Wright–Giemsa, etc.). The sputum may be obtained by induced cough procedures, fiberoptic bronchoscopy, and transbronchial biopsy. Consult an infectious disease specialist or pulmonologist.
2. Treat with trimethoprim-sulfamethoxazole (trimethoprim 15–20 mg/kg daily and sulfamethoxazole 75–100 mg/kg daily). This is given orally or by IV in four divided doses. Treatment is continued for 14 days.
3. Alternatively, pentamidine isethionate 4 mg/kg daily may be given as a single dose by slow IV infusion.
4. Consider corticosteroids in AIDS patients.

PNEUMONIA

1. Confirm diagnosis with sputum smear and culture, chest x-ray, cold agglutinins, and serologic tests of acute and convalescent sera.
2. *Bacterial pneumonia:*
   a. Treat initially with erythromycin 500 mg q.6h. or nafcillin 1 g q.4h.
   b. Once culture and sensitivity studies are back, treat accordingly.
3. *Mycoplasma pneumonia:* Treat with erythromycin 30−50 mg/kg daily in divided doses for 10−14 days. Alternatively, tetracycline 30−50 mg/kg daily may be given except in children under 8 years old.
4. *Legionnaires' disease:* Treat with erythromycin 500−1000 mg q.6h. or clarithromycin 750 mg q.12h. Rifampin may be added to the erythromycin in severe cases.
5. *Viral pneumonia:* Treatment is usually supportive. Ribavirin may be effective in RSV pneumonia, and amantadine HCl can be given for influenza pneumonia.

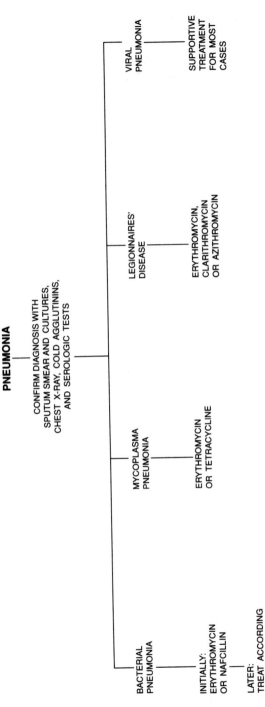

PNEUMONIA

CONFIRM DIAGNOSIS WITH
SPUTUM SMEAR AND CULTURES,
CHEST X-RAY, COLD AGGLUTININS,
AND SEROLOGIC TESTS

BACTERIAL
PNEUMONIA

INITIALLY:
ERYTHROMYCIN
OR NAFCILLIN

LATER:
TREAT ACCORDING
TO CULTURES
AND SENSITIVITIES

MYCOPLASMA
PNEUMONIA

ERYTHROMYCIN
OR TETRACYCLINE

LEGIONNAIRES'
DISEASE

ERYTHROMYCIN,
CLARITHROMYCIN
OR AZITHROMYCIN

VIRAL
PNEUMONIA

SUPPORTIVE
TREATMENT
FOR MOST
CASES

PNEUMOTHORAX

1. Confirm diagnosis by clinical examination and chest x-ray. Hospitalize patient.
2. *Spontaneous pneumothorax:*
   a. Less than 15%: Treat with observation.
   b. Moderate to severe: Try simple thoracentesis first. If that is unsuccessful, treat with tube thoracostomy. If that is unsuccessful, plan surgery (pleurodesis, pleurectomy, or surgical closure).
3. *Traumatic pneumothorax:* Tube thoracostomy; consult a thoracic surgeon.
4. *Tension pneumothorax:* Immediately insert a large bore needle into second anterior intercostal space. Follow with tube thoracostomy. Consult a thoracic surgeon as soon as possible.

PNEUMOTHORAX

CONFIRM DIAGNOSIS BY
CLINICAL EXAMINATION AND
CHEST X-RAY

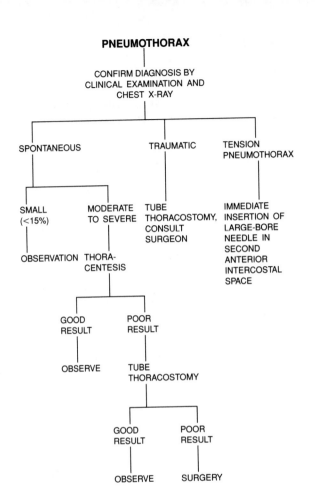

POLIOMYELITIS

1. Confirm diagnosis by clinical observation and spinal fluid analysis. Consult a neurologist.
2. Treatment is supportive. Respiratory support with respirator is the most important measure when indicated.
3. *Postpolio syndrome:* No treatment is available for this unfortunate delayed manifestation of the disease.

Prophylaxis

This is accomplished by oral polio vaccine in a series of three doses. The first two doses are given at 2 and 4 months, and the third dose is given at 15–18 months. Another dose is given just before entry into school.

POLYCYSTIC KIDNEY DISEASE

1. Confirm diagnosis by ultrasonography, intravenous pyelography, and CT scans. Consult a nephrologist. Screen members of family.
2. Treatment is primarily symptomatic. Recurrent urinary tract infections, hypertension, and renal failure must be addressed.
3. Occasionally, puncture of cysts and nephrectomy may be necessary. Consult a urologist.

POLYCYSTIC OVARY SYNDROME

1. Confirm diagnosis by clinical observation, elevated LH:FSH ratio, androstenedione and testosterone, and laparoscopy. Consult a gynecologist.
2. Weight reduction for all patients who are obese.
3. If patient desires to get pregnant, consider clomiphene administration or wedge resection of ovaries. Consult a gynecologist.
4. If patient is hirsute and does not desire pregnancy, administer oral contraceptives with both estrogen and progesterone components to control excess androgen. This will also help irregular menses.

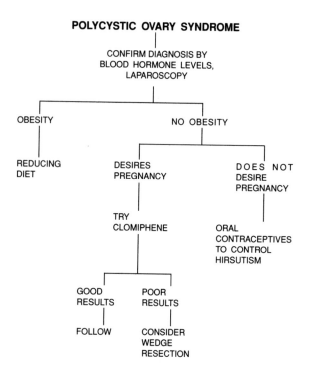

POLYCYTHEMIA VERA

1. Confirm diagnosis by findings of increased red cell mass, splenomegaly, thrombocytosis, and leukocytosis. Look for increased leukocyte alkaline phosphatase and elevated serum vitamin B_{12} levels.
2. Treat with frequent phlebotomy. If symptomatic iron deficiency develops, give iron supplement.
3. Hydroxyurea may be given, especially in elderly. Consult a hematologist or an oncologist.

POLYMYALGIA RHEUMATICA

1. Confirm diagnosis with marked elevation of sedimentation rate and temporal artery biopsy.
2. Treat with prednisone 10–15 mg/day initially. If results are poor, increase dose. Continue treatment for 4–8 weeks and then use maintenance dose of 5–10 mg to prevent relapse. Therapy may have to be continued for 2 years. Consult a rheumatologist in difficult cases.

PORPHYRIA

1. Confirm diagnosis by urine for porphyrins and porphobilinogens. δ-aminolevulinic acid is also increased.
2. Treatment is symptomatic. Intravenous heme may be tried. Consult a metabolic disease specialist.
3. Patients should avoid precipitating factors such as alcohol, barbiturates, many other anticonvulsants, sulfonamides, and estrogen-containing oral contraceptives. See standard textbooks for a more extensive listing of drugs to avoid.
4. Phlebotomy may be useful in porphyria cutanea tarda.

PREECLAMPSIA–ECLAMPSIA

1. Confirm diagnosis by observing for hypertension, edema, and proteinuria.
2. Consult an obstetrician.
3. Treat hypertension if diastolic blood pressure rises above 100 mm. Avoid alcohol and tobacco use. Administer methyldopa 250–500 mg t.i.d. orally or 500–1000 mg IV stat, followed by oral therapy. Administer hydralazine 25–75 mg b.i.d. to q.i.d. orally.
4. For convulsions and prevention of convulsions administer magnesium sulfate 4–6 g stat and 2 g/hour after that. Monitor blood every 4–6 hours to keep level at 5–7 mEq/100 cc. If convulsions continue to occur, give diazepam 5–10 mg IV. Treat overdose of magnesium sulfate with 10% calcium gluconate 10 ml IV.

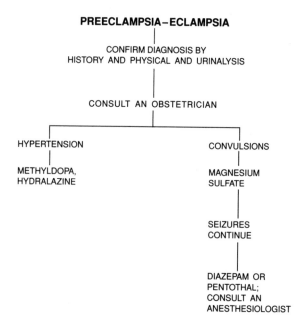

PREECLAMPSIA–ECLAMPSIA

CONFIRM DIAGNOSIS BY
HISTORY AND PHYSICAL AND URINALYSIS

CONSULT AN OBSTETRICIAN

HYPERTENSION

METHYLDOPA,
HYDRALAZINE

CONVULSIONS

MAGNESIUM
SULFATE

SEIZURES
CONTINUE

DIAZEPAM OR
PENTOTHAL;
CONSULT AN
ANESTHESIOLOGIST

PREMENSTRUAL TENSION SYNDROME

1. Confirm diagnosis by clinical evaluation.
2. First line of therapy is NSAIDs such as naproxen 250–375 mg t.i.d.
3. If the above are ineffective, a diuretic such as hydrochlorothiazide 25–50 mg/day or spironolactone 25 mg t.i.d. may be tried.
4. If the above are ineffective, low-dose oral contraceptives may prove beneficial. These include Loestrin 1/20 and Ortho-Novum 1/50. Consult a gynecologist.

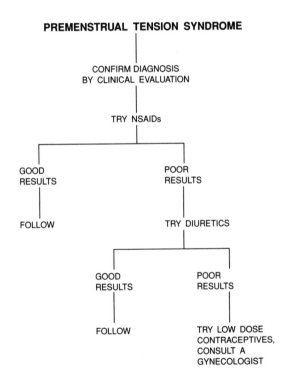

PROSTATIC CARCINOMA

1. Confirm diagnosis by transrectal ultrasonography, needle biopsy, serum prostate specific antigen (PSA), and acid and alkaline phosphatase. Consult a urologist and an oncologist.

2. *Stage A (clinically undetectable):* If patient is under 60 years of age, consider radical prostatectomy. If patient is over 70 years of age, observation may be the best course.

3. *Stage B (clinically detectable but restricted to the prostate):* If patient is under 60 consider radical prostatectomy, followed by radiation. If patient is over 60 years of age, external beam radiation is the treatment of choice.

4. *Stage C (localized tumor that has penetrated the prostate capsule):* External beam radiation is the treatment of choice.

5. *Stage D (metastasis to lymph nodes, bone, etc., or persistently elevated acid phosphatase):* Treat with hormonal manipulation in most cases, but external beam radiation may be tried in some cases.

PROSTATIC CARCINOMA

CONFIRM DIAGNOSIS BY
ULTRASONOGRAPHY, NEEDLE BIOPSY
AND SERUM PROSTATE SPECIFIC ANTIGEN (PSA).
CONSULT A UROLOGIST AND AN ONCOLOGIST

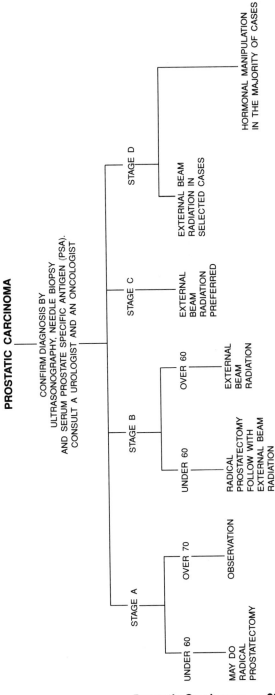

STAGE A

UNDER 60 — MAY DO RADICAL PROSTATECTOMY

OVER 70 — OBSERVATION

STAGE B

UNDER 60 — RADICAL PROSTATECTOMY FOLLOW WITH EXTERNAL BEAM RADIATION

OVER 60 — EXTERNAL BEAM RADIATION

STAGE C

EXTERNAL BEAM RADIATION PREFERRED

STAGE D

EXTERNAL BEAM RADIATION IN SELECTED CASES

HORMONAL MANIPULATION IN THE MAJORITY OF CASES

Prostatic Carcinoma 383

PROSTATIC HYPERTROPHY

1. Confirm diagnosis by history and physical examination, catheterization for residual urine, intravenous pyelography, and biopsy of the prostate. Cystoscopy and ultrasonography may be necessary. Consult a urologist.

2. *No obstructive symptoms:* These cases may be observed with frequent digital rectal examinations.

3. *Obstructive symptoms:*

   a. Mild with minimal residual urine: These patients deserve a trial of medical therapy with alpha-adrenergic antagonists (such as Hytrin 1–5 mg q.d.), finasteride, or luteinizing hormone-releasing hormone (LHRH). If results are poor, surgery should be considered.

   b. Moderate to severe: If there is only moderate enlargement of the gland, consider transurethral prostatectomy (TUR). If the gland is massively enlarged, open prostatectomy should be considered.

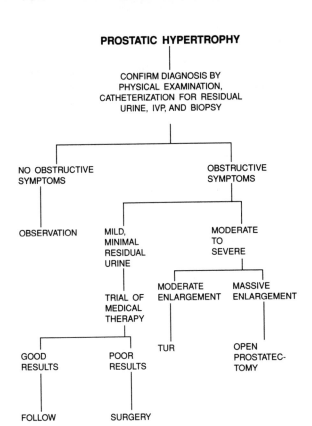

PROSTATIC HYPERTROPHY

CONFIRM DIAGNOSIS BY
PHYSICAL EXAMINATION,
CATHETERIZATION FOR RESIDUAL
URINE, IVP, AND BIOPSY

NO OBSTRUCTIVE
SYMPTOMS

OBSTRUCTIVE
SYMPTOMS

OBSERVATION

MILD,
MINIMAL
RESIDUAL
URINE

MODERATE
TO
SEVERE

MODERATE
ENLARGEMENT

MASSIVE
ENLARGEMENT

TRIAL OF
MEDICAL
THERAPY

TUR

OPEN
PROSTATEC-
TOMY

GOOD
RESULTS

POOR
RESULTS

FOLLOW

SURGERY

PROSTATITIS

1. Confirm diagnosis by urinalysis, urine cultures, and smear of fluid obtained from urethra after prostatic massage. Consult a urologist in difficult cases. Be sure to rule out gonorrhea.
2. Treat with doxycycline 100 mg b.i.d. for 3–4 weeks or trimethoprim-sulfamethoxazole (160–800 mg) b.i.d. for 30 days. In chronic cases, it may be necessary to continue treatment for 6 months. Prostatic massage may be helpful.

PSEUDOGOUT

1. Confirm diagnosis by examining synovial fluid for weakly positive birefringent crystals (calcium pyrophosphate crystals).
2. Treat with NSAIDs such as ibuprofen 800 mg t.i.d. or intra-articular corticosteroids such as 40 mg of triamcinolone acetate in 3–4 cc of 1% Xylocaine.
3. Prophylactic colchicine 0.6 mg b.i.d. may be helpful.

PSEUDOHYPOPARATHYROIDISM

1. Confirm diagnosis by family history, serum calcium and phosphorus levels, serum parathyroid hormone levels, and response of blood and urine calcium to exogenous parathyroid hormone.
2. Treat with vitamin D or calcitriol and high doses of oral calcium lactate or gluconate.

PSEUDO-PSEUDOHYPOPARATHYROIDISM

1. Confirm diagnosis by family history and clinical evaluation with (a) normal serum calcium and phosphorus levels and (b) normal response of urinary cyclic AMP to exogenous parathyroid hormone.
2. No treatment is necessary.

PSEUDOTUMOR CEREBRI

1. Confirm diagnosis by CT scans of the brain and lumbar puncture. Consult a neurologist.
2. Treat medically with weight reduction, diuretics (acetazolamide or furosemide), and dexamethasone in selected cases.
3. When there is increasing headache and visual disturbances despite medical therapy, consider a CSF shunting procedure. Consult a neurosurgeon.

PSITTACOSIS

1. Confirm diagnosis by sputum or blood culture and serologic tests (serologic tests are preferred).
2. Treat with tetracycline 500 mg q.6h. for 10–14 days or erythromycin 500 mg q.6h. for 10–14 days. Hospitalization may be indicated in severe cases.

PSORIASIS

1. Confirm diagnosis by family history, physical examination, and skin biopsy. Consult a dermatologist.
2. *Mild localized disease:* Treat with topical corticosteroids such as triamcinolone acetonide 0.1% ointment or cream. Cover the treatment areas with Saran wrap at night to provide more effective absorption.
3. *Mild to moderate generalized disease:* Whole-body ultraviolet B three to five times a week for 4–6 weeks. Alternatively, topical tar therapy may be used alone or in conjunction with the ultraviolet B.
4. *Severe generalized disease:* Treat with combined Psoralens and ultraviolet A radiation two to four times a week. Methotrexate may also be used. Consult a dermatologist.

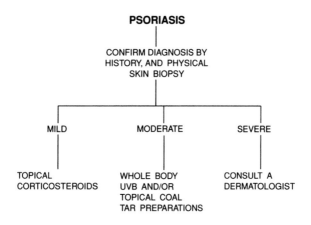

PULMONARY ALVEOLAR PROTEINOSIS

1. Confirm diagnosis by chest x-ray and lung biopsy.
2. Treat with whole-lung lavage. Consult a pulmonologist.

PULMONARY EMBOLISM

1. Confirm diagnosis by chest x-ray, ventilation–perfusion scans, or pulmonary angiography (if patient is unstable). Monitor arterial blood gases.
2. *If patient is stable:* Treat with hospitalization, 6 liters of oxygen by nasal cannula, IV fluids, and anticoagulation with heparin by continuous infusion. Watch for complications.
3. *If patient is unstable and exhibits significant hypotension, cor pulmonale, or both:* Hospitalize for pulmonary angiography; if a massive embolism is verified, start thrombolytic therapy (such as streptokinase). Consult a pulmonologist.
4. *If patient continues unstable despite thrombolytic therapy:* Consult cardiovascular surgeon for immediate embolectomy.

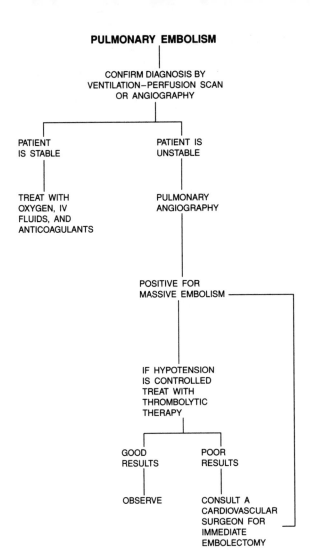

PULMONARY EMBOLISM

CONFIRM DIAGNOSIS BY
VENTILATION–PERFUSION SCAN
OR ANGIOGRAPHY

PATIENT
IS STABLE

PATIENT IS
UNSTABLE

TREAT WITH
OXYGEN, IV
FLUIDS, AND
ANTICOAGULANTS

PULMONARY
ANGIOGRAPHY

POSITIVE FOR
MASSIVE EMBOLISM

IF HYPOTENSION
IS CONTROLLED
TREAT WITH
THROMBOLYTIC
THERAPY

GOOD
RESULTS

POOR
RESULTS

OBSERVE

CONSULT A
CARDIOVASCULAR
SURGEON FOR
IMMEDIATE
EMBOLECTOMY

Pulmonary Embolism   395

PYELONEPHRITIS

1. Confirm diagnosis with urinalysis, urine culture and sensitivity, and colony count. Rule out various causes by intravenous pyelography and cystoscopy, especially in recurrent cases. Rule out systemic disease such as diabetes mellitus.
2. Initially, treat with trimethoprim-sulfamethoxazole (160 and 800 mg, respectively) twice daily for 14 days. Adjust therapy according to culture and sensitivity results.
3. Alternatively, a cephalosporin or fluoroquinolone may be used initially, especially in patients who are allergic to sulfa.

PYLORIC STENOSIS, CONGENITAL

1. Confirm diagnosis by history and physical examination and serum electrolytes. Consult a general surgeon.
2. Treat with surgery as soon as electrolytes are back in balance.

PYRIDOXINE DEFICIENCY

1. Confirm diagnosis by history, physical, and nerve conduction velocity studies.
2. Treat with pyridoxine 100 mg t.i.d. and multivitamin supplements.
3. Caution: Pyridoxine overdose may cause neuropathy also.

Q-FEVER

1. Confirm diagnosis by chest x-ray and serologic tests.
2. Treat with either chloramphenicol 50 mg/kg daily or tetracycline 25 mg/kg daily in four divided doses. Treatment is usually continued for 2 weeks.
3. Endocarditis requires prolonged antibiotic therapy.

RABIES

1. Confirm diagnosis by clinical picture, fluorescent antibody staining of tissue (corneal impression smears, skin or brain biopsy), and serologic tests.
2. Capture and isolate animal for 10 days. If any illness develops, sacrifice the animal and study tissue for rabies. If found, treat patient with postexposure prophylaxis.
3. If animal cannot be found and rabies is suspected in the area or species, treat with postexposure prophylaxis.
4. *Postexposure prophylaxis:*
   a. Scrub and clean wound.
   b. Administer human rabies immunoglobulin 20 units/kg one-half in the wound and the rest IM.
   c. Administer antirabies vaccine (HDCV).
5. Administer vaccine to individuals with high risk of contact with rabies (veterinarians, laboratory workers, etc.).

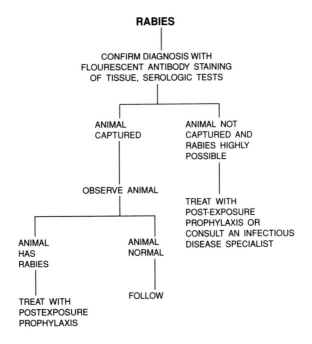

RAT-BITE FEVER

1. Confirm diagnosis by dark-field examination (Spirillum minus), cultures of blood or infected tissue *(Streptobacillus moniliformis),* or animal inoculation.
2. Treat with procaine penicillin 600,000 units IM b.i.d. for 2 weeks.
3. Alternatively, tetracycline 500 mg q.i.d. for 2 weeks may be utilized.

RAYNAUD'S DISEASE

1. Confirm diagnosis by history and physical examination and exclusion of all other causes of Raynaud's phenomena.
2. Treat with nifedipine 10–30 mg t.i.d. or diltiazem 30–90 mg t.i.d.
3. Alternatively, reserpine or prazosin may be tried.
4. Thoracic sympathectomy may be indicated in severe cases.

REFLEX SYMPATHETIC DYSTROPHY

1. Confirm diagnosis by clinical findings, x-rays of the involved extremities, and response to stellate ganglion or lumbar paravertebral block. Consult a neurologist or an anesthesiologist.
2. Treat with stellate ganglion or lumbar paravertebral block.
3. If results are good but not sustained, consider surgical sympathectomy. Consult a thoracic surgeon.
4. Occasionally, short courses of high-dose corticosteroids may be useful. Give prednisone at 60 mg/day for 4 days and gradually taper over 3–4 weeks.

REFLUX ESOPHAGITIS

1. Confirm diagnosis with barium swallow and upper GI series, esophagoscopy and biopsy, or pH monitoring.
2. *Conservative measures:* Avoid caffeine, cigarettes, alcohol, and fatty foods and lose weight. Elevate the head of the bed. Use antacids, bismuth, and alginate preparations for acute episodes.
3. If symptoms persist, try H2-receptor antagonists such as cimetidine 400 mg q.12h. or ranitidine 150 mg q.12h.
4. If symptoms persist, try omeprazole 20–40 mg/day or metoclopramide 10 mg q.8h.
5. When all types of medical therapy have failed, surgery is indicated. Consult a general surgeon to help determine which procedure (Nissen fundoplication, Hill repair, Belsey repair, etc.) is best for your patient.
6. *Complications:*
   a. Stricture is treated with dilatation or surgery.
   b. Barrett's esophagitis should be followed with repeated esophagoscopy.

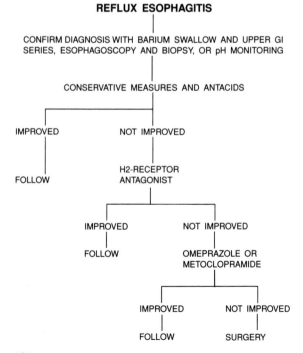

REFLUX ESOPHAGITIS

CONFIRM DIAGNOSIS WITH BARIUM SWALLOW AND UPPER GI SERIES, ESOPHAGOSCOPY AND BIOPSY, OR pH MONITORING

CONSERVATIVE MEASURES AND ANTACIDS

IMPROVED — NOT IMPROVED

FOLLOW

H2-RECEPTOR ANTAGONIST

IMPROVED — NOT IMPROVED

FOLLOW

OMEPRAZOLE OR METOCLOPRAMIDE

IMPROVED — NOT IMPROVED

FOLLOW — SURGERY

REFSUM'S DISEASE

1. Confirm diagnosis by finding elevated plasma phytanic acid and pipecolic acid.
2. Treat with chlorophyll-free diet and plasmapheresis in severe disease. Consult a neurologist and a hematologist.

REGIONAL ENTERITIS

1. Confirm diagnosis by small bowel series, barium enema, and colonoscopy and biopsy. Exploratory laparotomy may be necessary.
2. Treat mild to moderate cases with sulfasalazine 4–6 g/day.
3. In more severe cases, prednisone 45–60 mg/day may be added for 2–3 weeks and gradually tapered. Consult a gastroenterologist.
4. With small intestine involvement, obstruction may occur, requiring surgical intervention. Consult a general surgeon.
5. Parenteral alimentation may be necessary in severe cases. Consult a gastroenterologist.

REITER'S SYNDROME

1. Confirm diagnosis by clinical evaluation.
2. Treat first with NSAIDs such as indomethacin 25–50 mg t.i.d.
3. If the above treatment fails, azathioprine or methotrexate may be tried. Consult a rheumatologist.
4. Uveitis may require local and systemic corticosteroids. Consult an ophthalmologist.

RELAPSING FEVER

1. Confirm diagnosis by staining of peripheral blood films.
2. Treat with a single dose of oral or IV tetracycline 500 mg. For tick-borne infection, continue the tetracycline 500 mg q.i.d. for 10 days. Alternatively, erythromycin may be used.
3. Watch for Jarisch–Herxheimer reaction.

RELAPSING POLYCHONDRITIS

1. Confirm diagnosis by clinical observations and biopsy of cartilage.
2. Treat with prednisone 40–60 mg/day for 3–4 weeks and gradually taper. Cytotoxic agents may be tried if corticosteroids are ineffective. Consult a rheumatologist or an oncologist.

RENAL FAILURE, ACUTE

1. Confirm diagnosis with CBC, chemistry panel, electrolytes, and serum and urine osmolality. Renal biopsy later. Consult a nephrologist.
2. Catheterize for residual urine.
   a. Little or no urine: This indicates renal or pre-renal azotemia.
   b. Large volume of urine: This indicates postrenal azotemia or obstructive uropathy. The patient should be referred to a urologist.
3. Administer IV fluids and 25 g of mannitol.
   a. Good response: The patient probably has prerenal azotemia. Continue IV fluids, and monitor electrolytes and intake and output. Look for cause.
   b. Poor response: The patient has renal azotemia. Consult a nephrologist.
4. Treat the complications of renal azotemia
   a. Hyponatremia: Restrict fluids, monitor I&O, watch blood volume.
   b. Azotemia: Restrict protein intake. Give at least 100–200 g of glucose daily to restrict protein breakdown.
   c. Hyperkalemia: This is the most serious electrolyte disturbance. If it is mild, Kayexalate enemas may be sufficient. Glucose and insulin may give temporary relief. If it is severe, hemodialysis or peritoneal dialysis is indicated.
   d. Acidosis: If this is mild, oral bicarbonate may be given. If it is severe, hemodialysis or peritoneal dialysis must be done.
   e. Take precautions against infection.
   f. Remember to reduce drug dosage to compensate for reduced drug excretion via kidney.

RENAL FAILURE, ACUTE

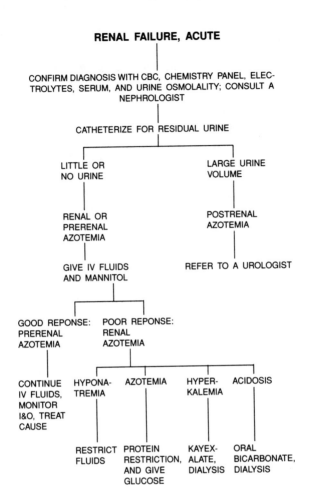

CONFIRM DIAGNOSIS WITH CBC, CHEMISTRY PANEL, ELEC-
TROLYTES, SERUM, AND URINE OSMOLALITY; CONSULT A
NEPHROLOGIST

CATHETERIZE FOR RESIDUAL URINE

LITTLE OR NO URINE

LARGE URINE VOLUME

RENAL OR PRERENAL AZOTEMIA

POSTRENAL AZOTEMIA

GIVE IV FLUIDS AND MANNITOL

REFER TO A UROLOGIST

GOOD REPONSE: PRERENAL AZOTEMIA

POOR REPONSE: RENAL AZOTEMIA

CONTINUE IV FLUIDS, MONITOR I&O, TREAT CAUSE

HYPONA-TREMIA

AZOTEMIA

HYPER-KALEMIA

ACIDOSIS

RESTRICT FLUIDS

PROTEIN RESTRICTION, AND GIVE GLUCOSE

KAYEX-ALATE, DIALYSIS

ORAL BICARBONATE, DIALYSIS

RENAL FAILURE, CHRONIC

1. Confirm diagnosis by CBC, chemistry panel, electrolytes, serum and urine osmolality and renal biopsy. Consult a nephrologist.
2. *Mild renal failure:*
   a. Hyponatremia: May need to restrict fluids or slightly increase sodium intake. Monitor I&O.
   b. Azotemia: Restrict protein to 1 g/kg daily.
   c. Hyperkalemia: This usually occurs only late in the course. It is a clear indication that dialysis must be started.
   d. Acidosis: This can be treated with oral bicarbonate.
   e. Hyperphosphatemia: Treat with oral phosphate binders such as calcium acetate or carbonate.
3. *Moderate to severe:*
   a. Hemodialysis or peritoneal dialysis must be started.
   c. Consider a renal transplant.

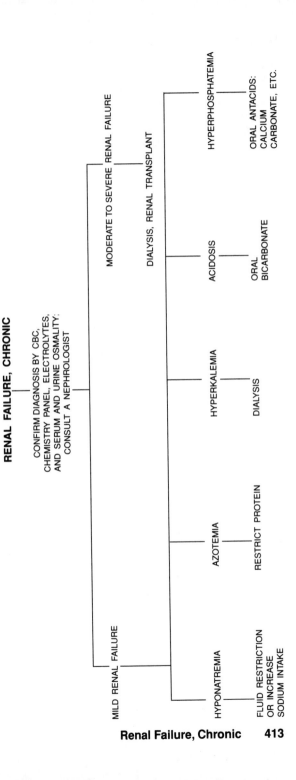

RENAL FAILURE, CHRONIC

CONFIRM DIAGNOSIS BY CBC, CHEMISTRY PANEL, ELECTROLYTES, AND SERUM AND URINE OSMALITY; CONSULT A NEPHROLOGIST

MILD RENAL FAILURE

MODERATE TO SEVERE RENAL FAILURE

DIALYSIS, RENAL TRANSPLANT

HYPONATREMIA

FLUID RESTRICTION OR INCREASE SODIUM INTAKE

AZOTEMIA

RESTRICT PROTEIN

HYPERKALEMIA

DIALYSIS

ACIDOSIS

ORAL BICARBONATE

HYPERPHOSPHATEMIA

ORAL ANTACIDS: CALCIUM CARBONATE, ETC.

RENAL VEIN THROMBOSIS

1. Confirm diagnosis by selective renal venography.
2. Treat with anticoagulants and thrombolytic therapy (streptokinase). Consult a nephrologist for guidance.
3. Thrombectomy and nephrectomy may be necessary in some cases. Consult a urologist.

RETINAL ARTERY OCCLUSION

1. Confirm diagnosis by clinical evaluation and retinoscopy. Consult an ophthalmologist.
2. Massage the eyeball to dislodge the embolism and have patient rebreathe into a paper bag to raise the CO_2 level in the blood.
3. An ophthalmologist will perform anterior chamber paracentesis.

RHEUMATIC FEVER

1. Confirm diagnosis with streptococcal antibody tests (such as ASO titer), sedimentation rate, and CRP.
2. Eliminate streptococcal infection with 1.2 million units of benzathine penicillin IM. Use erythromycin for penicillin-sensitive individuals.
3. Treat polyarthritis with aspirin 100−125 mg/kg daily.
4. For persistent carditis, add corticosteroids (such as prednisone 60−120 mg/day in four divided doses). Continue treatment until sedimentation rate is normal and then gradually taper, preventing rebound by overlapping with aspirin therapy. Consult a cardiologist or pediatrician for guidance.
5. Salicylates and corticosteroids have no effect on chorea.
6. Prevention by early treatment of streptococcal pharyngitis (see page 357).

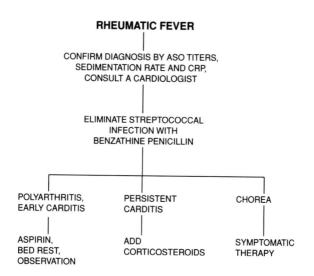

RHEUMATIC FEVER

CONFIRM DIAGNOSIS BY ASO TITERS, SEDIMENTATION RATE AND CRP, CONSULT A CARDIOLOGIST

ELIMINATE STREPTOCOCCAL INFECTION WITH BENZATHINE PENICILLIN

POLYARTHRITIS, EARLY CARDITIS	PERSISTENT CARDITIS	CHOREA
ASPIRIN, BED REST, OBSERVATION	ADD CORTICOSTEROIDS	SYMPTOMATIC THERAPY

RHEUMATOID ARTHRITIS

1. Confirm diagnosis by clinical observation, sedimentation rate, positive titer for rheumatoid factor, x-rays, and synovial analysis.
2. *Juvenile rheumatoid arthritis:*
   a. With systemic involvement (Still's disease): Corticosteroids such as prednisone 0.5–1.0 mg/kg daily as a single dose. This may be given daily or on alternate days until the disease is brought under control and then tapered. Intravenous "pulse" methylprednisolone may also be used. Consult a rheumatologist.
   b. Without significant systemic involvement: Treat as adult form of the disease.
3. *Adult rheumatoid arthritis:*
   a. First line of defense includes aspirin (in doses adequate to keep serum salicylate levels at 20–30 mg/dl) and other NSAIDs. Ibuprofen is given in doses of 400–800 mg t.i.d. Naproxen is given in doses of 250–500 mg t.i.d. Piroxicam is given at 20 mg/day. Ketoprofen is given at 100–300 mg/day.
   b. If NSAIDs are ineffective, a rheumatologist should be consulted to consider a disease-modifying antirheumatoid agent. Gold salts may be given or triethylphosphine 0.1–0.2 mg/kg daily. Sulfasalazine may be given in doses of 40–50 mg/kg daily in three to four divided doses. D-Penicillamine is given in doses of 5 mg/kg daily, up to 750 mg one day. Follow manufacturer's recommendation for monitoring laboratory studies with these drugs to avoid toxicity.
   c. If the above drugs are ineffective, an immunosuppressant such as methotrexate (7.5–15 mg once a week) or cyclophosphamide 1–2 mg/kg daily may be tried. Again, a rheumatologist should be consulted.
   d. Intra-articular corticosteroids given in localized flare-ups of the disease, especially in large joints. Triamcinolone diacetate 5–40 mg in saline or lidocaine 1% mixture is very effective.

e. Surgery, particularly total replacement of a number of joints, can be very successful. Consult an orthopedic surgeon.

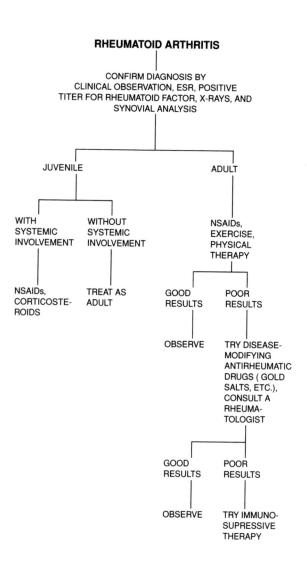

RHEUMATOID ARTHRITIS

CONFIRM DIAGNOSIS BY
CLINICAL OBSERVATION, ESR, POSITIVE
TITER FOR RHEUMATOID FACTOR, X-RAYS, AND
SYNOVIAL ANALYSIS

JUVENILE

WITH SYSTEMIC INVOLVEMENT

NSAIDs, CORTICOSTE-ROIDS

WITHOUT SYSTEMIC INVOLVEMENT

TREAT AS ADULT

ADULT

NSAIDs, EXERCISE, PHYSICAL THERAPY

GOOD RESULTS

OBSERVE

POOR RESULTS

TRY DISEASE-MODIFYING ANTIRHEUMATIC DRUGS (GOLD SALTS, ETC.), CONSULT A RHEUMA-TOLOGIST

GOOD RESULTS

OBSERVE

POOR RESULTS

TRY IMMUNO-SUPRESSIVE THERAPY

RHEUMATOID SPONDYLITIS

1. Confirm diagnosis by x-rays of the lumbar spine, bone scans, and finding of histocompatability antigen HLA-B27.
2. Treat with exercise, physiotherapy, and NSAIDs. Phenylbutazone is the most effective NSAID. The dose is 100–300 mg day. Sulfasalazine 500 mg q.6h. may also be effective.
3. Radiation therapy is occasionally indicated.
4. Consult an orthopedic surgeon if total hip arthroplasty becomes necessary.
5. Corticosteroids may be necessary when there is systemic involvement (uveitis, etc.).

RIBOFLAVIN DEFICIENCY

1. Confirm diagnosis by clinical findings (stomatitis, cheilosis, etc.) and response to therapy.
2. Treat with 5 mg riboflavin t.i.d. and multiple vitamins, as well.

RICKETS

1. Confirm diagnosis by serum and urine calcium, alkaline phosphatase, and skeletal survey.
2. Treat with oral vitamin D2 or D3 800–4000 IU (international units) daily for 6–12 weeks, followed by a maintenance dose of 400 IU (international units) daily. For good results, the diet must be adequate in calcium and phosphorus.

RICKETTSIALPOX

1. Confirm diagnosis with Weil–Felix reaction (usually negative) and serologic tests such as the complement-fixation test.
2. Treat with tetracycline 25 mg/kg daily or chloramphenicol 50 mg/kg daily in divided doses. Continue antibiotics for 24–48 hours after patient is afebrile, depending on the general improvement of the patient.

ROCKY MOUNTAIN SPOTTED FEVER

1. Confirm diagnosis with Weil–Felix reaction and specific serologic tests such as the complement-fixation test.
2. Treat with tetracycline 25 mg/kg daily or chloramphenicol 50 mg/kg daily in divided doses. Continue antibiotics until patient is afebrile and stable at least 24–48 hours.

RUBELLA

1. Confirm diagnosis by the clinical picture. Serologic tests are available for detection in confusing cases.
2. No specific therapy is available, but gamma globulin can abort the clinical symptomatology. Transfer of the disease from mother to fetus can still occur, even with gamma globulin administration.
3. *Prophylaxis:* This is obtained by giving MMR (measles–mumps–rubella) vaccine at 15 months of age or older. Lifetime immunity is probably conferred on most recipients. The vaccine cannot be given to pregnant women or any woman who expects to become pregnant within 3 months of receiving the vaccine.

RUBEOLA

1. Confirm diagnosis by clinical picture and stains of nasal secretions, sputum, and urine for multi-nucleated giant cells. Complement-fixation and other serologic tests are available.
2. There is no specific treatment. The disease can be modified or prevented with gamma globulin 0.25 ml/kg if given within 6 days of exposure.
3. *Prophylaxis:* MMR (measles–mumps–rubella) vaccine given at 15 months of age confers immunity for 20 years or more.

SALMONELLOSIS

1. Confirm diagnosis by stool cultures for enteric pathogens and serologic tests. Consult an infectious disease specialist.
2. *Enterocolitis:*
   a. High-risk patients (elderly, neonates, AIDS patients, etc.): Treat with chloramphenicol 50 mg/kg daily or ampicillin 150–200 mg/kg daily parenterally until afebrile and then orally for 2 weeks.
   b. Other patients: Treatment unnecessary.
   c. Treat electrolyte imbalance.
3. *Bacteremia and focal infections (infected aneurysm, osteomyelitis, etc.):* Treat with antibiotics as above plus surgical excision where indicated. Consult an infectious disease specialist.
4. *Enteric fever:* Treat with antibiotics as above. Trimethoprim 5 mg/kg q.12h. and sulfamethoxazole 25 mg/kg q.12h may be given parenterally and then continued orally after patient becomes afebrile.
5. *Carrier state:* Treat with ampicillin or amoxicillin 4–6 g/day in divided doses for 4–6 weeks. Trimethoprim 160 mg and sulfamethoxazole 800 mg q.12h. is also effective. Cholecystectomy may be necessary.

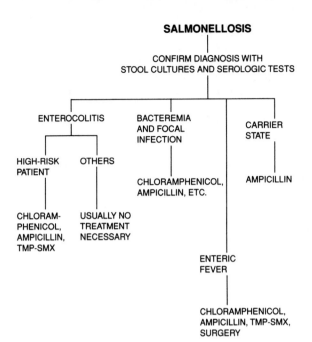

SALPINGITIS

1. Confirm diagnosis by vaginal or endocervical smear and culture, ultrasonography, endometrial biopsy, and laparoscopy. Look for tuberculosis in older women, especially.
2. Treat with doxycycline 100 mg q.12h. IV and cefotetan 2.0 g q.12h. IV. Continue for 48 hours after clinical improvement and then continue doxycycline 100 mg b.i.d. by mouth for 14 days total.
3. Alternatively, clindamycin may be given 800 mg q.8h. IV plus a loading dose of gentamicin 2.0 mg/kg and then 1.5 mg/kg q.8h IV. Continue these drugs until the patient is improved for 48 hours and then discharge on doxycycline 100 mg b.i.d. for 14 days total.

SARCOIDOSIS

1. Confirm diagnosis by chest x-ray, scalene node or transbronchial biopsy, the Kveim–Siltzbach skin test, and the clinical picture. Consult a pulmonologist.
2. Treat mild cases symptomatically.
3. Treat more severe cases, especially those with significant neurological, ocular, or cardiovascular involvement with prednisone 1 mg/kg day for 4–6 weeks and gradually taper over 8- to 12-week period. Consult a pulmonologist.

SCABIES

1. Confirm the diagnosis by microscopic examination of scrapings or biopsy of the burrows or papulovesicular lesions.
2. Treat with 5% permethrin cream applied over whole body from the neck down after bathing. Remove after 8 hours. Be sure to change the bed sheets before retiring again.
3. Alternatively, 1% lindane lotion may be used in the same manner. Beware of its neurotoxicity.

SCARLET FEVER

1. Confirm diagnosis by clinical picture, Dick test, and throat cultures.
2. Treat with penicillin V 250 mg p.o. q.i.d. for 10 days for adults and 125 mg q.i.d. for children less than 27 kg.
3. In patients suspected of poor compliance, give benzathine penicillin G 1.2 million units IM.
4. In patients with penicillin allergy, give erythromycin (10 mg/kg) up to 250 mg q.i.d. for 10 days. A first-generation cephalosporin may also be utilized.

SCHILDER'S DISEASE

1. Confirm diagnosis by MRI or CT scan of the brain, EEG, and spinal fluid analysis. Consult a neurologist.
2. Treatment is primarily supportive, but a course of corticosteroids or ACTH may be tried.

SCHISTOSOMIASIS

1. Confirm diagnosis by finding eggs in stools, urine, and tissues. Ultrasonography of the liver is helpful. Consult an infectious disease specialist.
2. *Schistosoma hematobium:* Treat with single dose of praziquantel 40 mg/kg or metrifonate 7.5–10 mg/kg given every other week for three doses.
3. *Schistosoma mansoni:* Treat with oxamniquine 15 mg/kg as a single dose with food or praziquantel 40 mg/kg as a single dose with food or as two divided doses 4 hours apart with food. Higher doses may be necessary in Africa and the Middle East. Praziquantel is the preferred drug in Africa.
4. *Schistosoma japonicum:* Treat with praziquantel 20 mg/kg q.4h. with food for three doses.

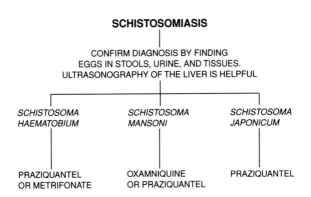

SCHIZOPHRENIA

1. Confirm diagnosis by clinical picture and psychometric testing. Consult a psychiatrist.
2. Treat with butyrophenones, phenothiazines, and dibenzodiazepines. Consult a psychiatrist for guidance in selection of drugs and dosage.

SCLERODERMA

1. Confirm diagnosis by clinical picture, antinuclear antibody titer, antinucleolar antibody titer, and other serologic tests. Skin biopsy may be helpful. Consult a rheumatologist.
2. No specific therapy is available, but D-penicillamine, corticosteroids, and various immunosuppressants may be tried under the guidance of a rheumatologist.
3. Treat reflux esophagitis with the usual measures (page 404).

SCRUB TYPHUS

1. Confirm diagnosis by the Weil–Felix reaction and other serologic tests.
2. Treat with tetracycline 25 mg/kg daily until the patient has been clinically improved and afebrile for 24–72 hours.
3. Alternatively, chloramphenicol 50 mg/kg daily may be given in like manner.

SCURVY

1. Confirm diagnosis by clinical picture, capillary fragility testing, and platelet ascorbic acid levels.
2. Treat with ascorbic acid 100 mg q.i.d. for 10 days and then 100 mg/day. Supplement with a well-balanced diet.

SEBORRHEIC DERMATITIS

1. Confirm diagnosis by clinical picture and skin biopsy.
2. Treat scalp involvement initially with a tar shampoo (T/Gel, etc.) or selenium sulfide shampoo (Selsun Gold). If this is not adequate, topical corticosteroids may be used, such as 0.1% triamcinolone (Kenalog) or fluocinonide 0.05% (Lidex). Apply once or twice a day. A shower cap may be applied overnight to increase the response to corticosteroids.
3. Involvement of the face is treated with low-potency corticosteroid cream, such as 1–2% hydrocortisone cream, desonide, or alclometasone dipropionate.
4. Treat areas of involvement other than the face with 0.1% triamcinolone or other medium-potency topical steroids. Topical ketoconazole cream may be effective.

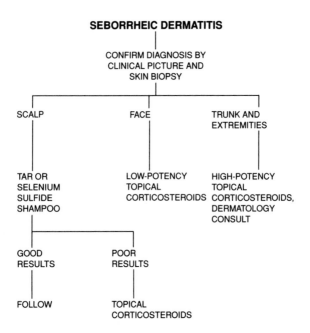

438

SEPTIC ARTHRITIS

1. Confirm diagnosis by smear and culture of synovial fluids and blood cultures.
2. Antibiotics are given according to smear and cultures. Ceftriaxone 2 g IV q.12h. may be given until a definitive organism is isolated. Consult an orthopedic surgeon.
3. Daily arthrocentesis should be performed until the synovial analysis is normal.

SEPTICEMIA

1. Confirm diagnosis by clinical picture and multiple blood cultures. Look for site of original infection. Consult an infectious disease expert.
2. Treat with cefotaxime 3 g IV q.6h. and gentamicin 1.5 mg/kg IV q.8h. until blood culture results are in or a focus of infection is established. If anaerobic infection is suspected, add clindamycin 600 mg IV q.6h. If *Staphylococcus* is suspected, use nafcillin 3 g IV q.6h. or vancomycin 15 mg/kg IV q.12h. When *Pseudomonas* infection is suspected, ceftazidime and tobramycin are utilized.

SERUM SICKNESS

1. Confirm diagnosis by history and physical, increased sedimentation rate and decreased serum complement. Consult an allergist.
2. Withdraw the offending agent.
3. If there is significant shock, patient should be hospitalized and treated with oxygen, intravenous fluids, and Solu-Cortef 200 mg q.6h. IV.
4. Mild to moderate disease may be treated with oral prednisone 1–2 mg/kg daily for 2–5 days and gradually tapering over 1- to 2-week period once the patient is asymptomatic.
5. Antihistamines will relieve the patient's pruritus, and NSAIDs will relieve the fever and arthralgias.

SHIGELLOSIS

1. Confirm diagnosis by stool smear and culture and serological tests when available.
2. Treat mild cases with oral rehydration (see page 82) or intravenous replacement fluids.
3. Moderate to severe cases can be treated with ampicillin 50–100 mg/kg daily in children, 2–4 g/day in adults, or trimethoprim-sulfamethoxazole 8/40 mg/kg daily in children or 160/800 mg q.12h. in adults.

SHY-DRAGER SYNDROME

1. Confirm diagnosis by the clinical picture and finding of a fall in systolic blood pressure of 30 mm or more in rising to the standing position and anhidrosis.
2. Treat postural hypotension with antigravity stockings and increased salt intake combined with fludrohydrocortisone 0.05–0.2 mg/day. Consult a cardiologist.
3. Treat Parkinson's syndrome with Sinemet or bromocriptine (page 338).

SICKLE CELL ANEMIA

1. Confirm diagnosis by sickle cell preps and hemoglobin electrophoresis.
2. No specific treatment is available. Nonspecific therapy such as increased folic acid intake, prompt treatment of infection, analgesics, and hydration for painful crisis and occasional blood transfusions have their place. Consult a hematologist for guidance.
3. Pneumococcal vaccine should be given to prevent pneumococcal sepsis.

SINUSITIS

1. Confirm diagnosis by transillumination, x-rays of sinuses, CT scan, and nose and throat cultures.
2. Treat with nasal decongestants, hydration, steam inhalation, and antibiotics. Amoxicillin 500 mg t.i.d., trimethoprim-sulfamethoxazole 160/800 mg b.i.d., or a second-generation cephalosporin may be used.
3. If the patient does not respond to the above measures within 24 hours, consider referral to an otolaryngologist for irrigation of the sinus involved.

SJÖGREN'S SYNDROME

1. Confirm diagnosis by the clinical picture and excluding other disorders. Consult a rheumatologist.
2. No specific treatment is available.
3. Treat the sicca complex with fluid replacement, artificial tears, and referral to an ophthalmologist if corneal ulcers develop.
4. Corticosteroids such as prednisone 1 mg/kg daily may be given to treat renal or other systemic involvement. Other immunosuppressant drugs may be used.

SKIN CANCER

1. Confirm diagnosis by skin biopsy.
2. Treat with surgery, radiation, or chemotherapy based on consultation with a dermatologist. Remember, squamous cell carcinoma can occasionally metastasize.

SLEEP APNEA

1. Confirm diagnosis by polysomnography. Consult a pulmonologist for guidance in diagnosis and treatment.
2. *Obstructive sleep apnea:*
   a. Treat initially with nasal continuous positive airway pressure (CPAP) during sleep. Weight reduction and avoidance of alcohol should be accomplished in all cases, if possible.
   b. Some patients may respond to tricyclic medication such as protriptyline 20–30 mg h.s.
   c. Some patients may benefit from uvulopalatopharyngoplasty. Consult an otolaryngologist for evaluation for this procedure.
3. *Central sleep apnea:*
   a. Patients with hypoxemia benefit from supplemental oxygen through the night.
   b. Some patients respond to acetazolamide.
   c. Some patients respond to CPAP.

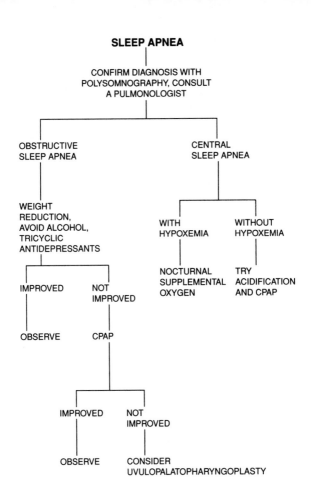

SLEEP APNEA

CONFIRM DIAGNOSIS WITH
POLYSOMNOGRAPHY, CONSULT
A PULMONOLOGIST

OBSTRUCTIVE
SLEEP APNEA

CENTRAL
SLEEP APNEA

WEIGHT
REDUCTION,
AVOID ALCOHOL,
TRICYCLIC
ANTIDEPRESSANTS

WITH
HYPOXEMIA

WITHOUT
HYPOXEMIA

NOCTURNAL
SUPPLEMENTAL
OXYGEN

TRY
ACIDIFICATION
AND CPAP

IMPROVED

NOT
IMPROVED

OBSERVE

CPAP

IMPROVED

NOT
IMPROVED

OBSERVE

CONSIDER
UVULOPALATOPHARYNGOPLASTY

SMALL INTESTINAL TUMORS

1. Confirm diagnosis by upper GI series and progress meal, CT scans with contrast, and exploratory laparotomy.
2. Consult general surgeon for resection.
3. Complications include intestinal obstruction, bleeding, and bowel perforation. All of these complications require immediate surgical consult.

SNAKE BITE

1. Confirm diagnosis by history and clinical picture.
2. Determine if envenomation took place and the size of the snake.
3. Patient is placed at rest, and the involved extremity is immobilized. A constrictive band is placed 1 inch above the bite to impede lymphatic flow. This is released if it becomes tight and then repositioned above the swelling. I&D and suction is no longer recommended.
4. Patient is transferred to a hospital where treatment of shock and respiratory difficulty can be instituted and appropriate antivenin given intravenously. Consult an expert in snake bites for further treatment. Polyvalent crotaline antivenin for all American pit vipers and the North American coral snake is commercially available.

SPASMODIC TORTICOLLIS

1. Confirm diagnosis by clinical evaluation.
2. Treat initially with gradually increasing doses of trihexyphenidyl and diazepam. May need to be as much as 80 mg/day.
3. Other drugs such as carbamazepine or haloperidol may be tried.
4. If the above measures are unsuccessful, injections of botulinum toxin may be tried. Consult a neurologist or someone with a lot of experience in their use.
5. In resistant cases, denervative surgical procedures may be tried. Consult a neurosurgeon.

SPINAL CORD TUMOR

1. Confirm diagnosis by MRIs and myelography combined with CT scans.
2. Consult a neurosurgeon for immediate surgical intervention. The role of radiation and chemotherapy is not well-defined. Consult an oncologist.

SPOROTRICHOSIS

1. Confirm diagnosis with culture of pus, synovial fluid, sputum, or skin biopsy.
2. *Cutaneous sporotrichosis:* Treat with saturated solution of potassium iodide up to 4.5–9 ml/day. Treat for 1 month after resolution.
3. Itraconazole may be tried in patients who are allergic to iodine.
4. *Extracutaneous sporotrichosis:* Treat with amphotericin B.

SPRAINS, COMMON

1. Confirm diagnosis by history and physical examination, x-rays, and occasionally MRIs to rule out more serious pathology.
2. *Cervical, thoracic, and lumbar sprains:*
   a. Treat initially with physiotherapy, cervical collar or lumbosacral support, anti-inflammatory drugs, muscle relaxants, and analgesics. Consider complete bed rest.
   b. If pain persists after 4–6 weeks, consider trigger point therapy, facet injections, and epidural blocks. Consider chiropractic.
   c. If pain persists, consider MRIs, electromyography, evoked potential, and nerve conduction velocity studies and referral to an orthopedic or neurological specialist.
3. *Wrist, knee, and ankle sprains:*
   a. Treat initially with rest, elevation, and Ace bandage. Cold packs are useful the first 24 hours and then warm packs.
   b. If pain persists, add anti-inflammatory drugs and physiotherapy.
   c. If pain persists, consider referral to orthopedic surgeon for casting and other diagnostic procedures.

SPRAINS, COMMON

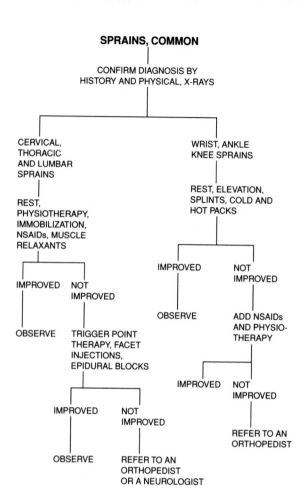

CONFIRM DIAGNOSIS BY
HISTORY AND PHYSICAL, X-RAYS

CERVICAL, THORACIC AND LUMBAR SPRAINS

REST, PHYSIOTHERAPY, IMMOBILIZATION, NSAIDs, MUSCLE RELAXANTS

IMPROVED → OBSERVE

NOT IMPROVED → TRIGGER POINT THERAPY, FACET INJECTIONS, EPIDURAL BLOCKS

IMPROVED → OBSERVE

NOT IMPROVED → REFER TO AN ORTHOPEDIST OR A NEUROLOGIST

WRIST, ANKLE KNEE SPRAINS

REST, ELEVATION, SPLINTS, COLD AND HOT PACKS

IMPROVED → OBSERVE

NOT IMPROVED → ADD NSAIDs AND PHYSIOTHERAPY

IMPROVED

NOT IMPROVED → REFER TO AN ORTHOPEDIST

STASIS DERMATITIS

1. Confirm diagnosis by clinical picture.
2. Treat with elevation of the legs, graded compression stockings, or support hose and corticosteroid creams or ointments.
3. Venous stripping and ligation may be necessary.

STRONGYLOIDIASIS

1. Confirm diagnosis by stool examinations for the larvae, examination of duodenal aspiration fluid, or Enterotest string method. Serologic tests are also available.
2. For most cases, thiabendazole 25 mg/kg is given b.i.d. for 2 days.
3. In disseminated strongyloidiasis, treatment is extended for 5–7 days. Do not discontinue the drug until the parasites are eradicated.

STURGE–WEBER SYNDROME

1. Confirm diagnosis by clinical picture and CT scans.
2. Treat seizures as with any form of epilepsy (page 140).
3. Intractable seizures may respond to resection of large blocks of the involved brain.

SUBACUTE BACTERIAL ENDOCARDITIS

1. Confirm diagnosis by serial blood cultures and echocardiography routine and transesophageal. Now techniques are available which can identify the organism immunologically without cultures. Consult a cardiologist.
2. Treat with 20 million units of penicillin G by continuous intravenous administration, along with gentamicin 1 mg/kg q.8h. Once cultures are back, use antibiotics according to the organism isolated. Determine minimum inhibitory concentration and minimum bacteriocidal concentration to determine exact dose.
3. After 2 weeks of IV therapy, the patient may be switched to oral antibiotics.
4. Alternatively, vancomycin 30 mg/kg/day or cephtriaxone 1–2 gm/day may be given.
5. Endocarditis due to staphylococcus aureus or epidermidis may be treated with nafcillin 2 gm q 4–6 hrs for 4–6 weeks and gentamicin 1 mg/kg/q 8 hrs for the first 3–5 days.

SUBDIAPHRAGMATIC ABSCESS

1. Confirm diagnosis by chest x-ray, flat plate of abdomen, ultrasonography, and CT scans.
2. Begin antibiotics, including a third-generation cephalosporin and gentamicin as soon as blood cultures have been obtained.
3. Consult a surgeon immediately for percutaneous or open drainage of abscess.

SUBDURAL HEMATOMA

1. Confirm diagnosis by CT scans or MRI.
2. Consult a neurosurgeon immediately for surgical evacuation. Small hematomas usually do not require therapy, but let the neurosurgeon decide that.

SYPHILIS

1. Confirm diagnosis by dark-field examination, direct fluorescent antibody identification test (DFA-TP), VDRL, or fluorescent treponemal antibody-absorption test (FTA-ABS). The latter test is especially useful for late syphilis.
2. *Primary, secondary, or early latent syphilis:* Treat with benzathine penicillin G 2.4 million units IM.
3. *Late latent syphilis, cardiovascular syphilis, or benign tertiary syphilis:*
   a. Do lumbar puncture.
   b. If lumbar puncture is normal, treat with benzathine penicillin G 2.4 million units IM weekly for 3 weeks.
   c. If lumbar puncture is abnormal, treat as neurosyphilis.
4. *Neurosyphilis:* Treat with aqueous penicillin G 12–14 million units a day IV for 14 days.
5. *Syphilis in pregnancy:* Treat according to stage.
6. For patients with penicillin allergy, use tetracycline 500 mg q.i.d. orally for 2 weeks for primary, secondary, or early latent syphilis, and extend it to 4 weeks in late latent syphilis. Patients with neurosyphilis should be desensitized to penicillin and treated with penicillin.

SYPHILIS

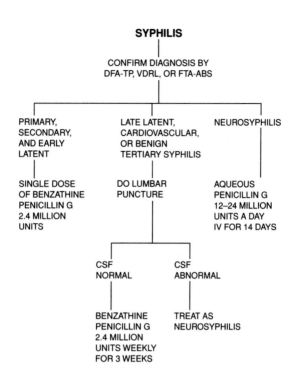

CONFIRM DIAGNOSIS BY
DFA-TP, VDRL, OR FTA-ABS

PRIMARY,
SECONDARY,
AND EARLY
LATENT

SINGLE DOSE
OF BENZATHINE
PENICILLIN G
2.4 MILLION
UNITS

LATE LATENT,
CARDIOVASCULAR,
OR BENIGN
TERTIARY SYPHILIS

DO LUMBAR
PUNCTURE

CSF
NORMAL

BENZATHINE
PENICILLIN G
2.4 MILLION
UNITS WEEKLY
FOR 3 WEEKS

CSF
ABNORMAL

TREAT AS
NEUROSYPHILIS

NEUROSYPHILIS

AQUEOUS
PENICILLIN G
12–24 MILLION
UNITS A DAY
IV FOR 14 DAYS

SYRINGOMYELIA

1. Confirm diagnosis by combined CT scan and myelography or MRI.
2. Consult a neurosurgeon for decompression of the cavity or other appropriate neurosurgical treatment.

SYSTEMIC MASTOCYTOSIS

1. Confirm diagnosis by 24-hour urine histamine, blood histamine level, and skin or bone marrow biopsy.
2. *Mild to moderate flushing and pruritus:* Treat with an H1 antihistamine.
3. *Gastric acid hypersecretion:* Treat with an H2 antihistamine or proton pump inhibitor.
4. *Diarrhea and abdominal pain:* Treat with cromolyn sodium.
5. *Severe flushing and vascular collapse:* Treat with NSAIDs.

TAKAYASU'S DISEASE

1. Confirm diagnosis by elevated sedimentation rate, protein electrophoresis, and arteriography. Consult a cardiovascular surgeon.
2. Treat systemic symptoms with corticosteroids such as prednisone 40–60 mg/day for 2–3 weeks and gradually taper.
3. Treat stenosed blood vessels with angiography and other surgical techniques. Consult a cardiovascular surgeon.

TAPEWORM DISEASE

1. Confirm diagnosis by stools for ovum and parasites, fluorescent antibody tests, tissue biopsy, x-rays, and CT scans.
2. Treat with praziquantel 20 mg/kg as a single dose.
3. Larval cysts can be excised surgically.

TEMPORAL ARTERITIS

1. Confirm diagnosis by high sedimentation rate and superficial temporal artery biopsy.
2. Treat with corticosteroids such as prednisone 60 mg/day and gradually tapering over a 4- to 6-week period. A maintenance dose of 7.5–10 mg is required for 1–2 years to prevent relapses.

TESTICULAR TUMORS

1. Confirm diagnosis with clinical evaluation, CT scan of the abdomen and pelvis, chest x-ray, alpha-fetoprotein, and human chorionic gonadotropin. Consult an oncologist.
2. *Early seminoma:* Treat with orchiectomy, followed by abdominal radiotherapy.
3. *Advanced seminoma:* Treat initially with combination chemotherapy. This may be followed by surgery, radiation, or further chemotherapy. Consult an oncologist for guidance.
4. *Nonseminoma stage I:* Treat with orchiectomy and retroperitoneal lymph node dissection or orchiectomy alone, followed by observation.
5. *Nonseminoma stage II:* Treatment is controversial. Consult an oncologist for guidance.
6. *Advanced nonseminoma:* Combined chemotherapy under the direction of an experienced oncologist offers the best survival rate.
7. Meticulous follow-up of all patients is mandatory.

TETANUS

1. Confirm diagnosis by the history of IV drug use and the clinical picture.
2. Treat the bacterial infection with 10–12 million units of aqueous penicillin G daily for 10 days. Alternative drugs are erythromycin and clindamycin.
3. Administer human tetanus immune globulin 3000–6000 units IM in divided doses.
4. Consult an anesthesiologist for intubation or tracheotomy and general anesthesia during the tetany. Diazepam and lorazepam are given for severe muscle spasm, as well as neuromuscular blockade.

THALASSEMIA

1. Confirm diagnosis by CBC, examination of peripheral blood smears, and hemoglobin electrophoresis.
2. Consult a hematologist for treatment with blood transfusions, bone marrow transplants, and desferrioxamine to remove excess iron.

THORACIC OUTLET SYNDROME

1. Confirm diagnosis by clinical picture, somatosensory evoked potential studies, and brachial angiography.
2. Treat with shoulder shrugs, exercise, and adjustment of posture.
3. Surgery may be considered if above treatment is unsuccessful. Consult an orthopedic surgeon or a neurosurgeon.

THROMBOANGIITIS OBLITERANS

1. Confirm diagnosis by arteriography and excisional biopsy.
2. No specific treatment is available.
3. Stop smoking.
4. Surgical treatment includes arterial bypass, local débridement, and amputation of involved extremity.

THROMBOCYTOPENIA PURPURA, IDIOPATHIC

1. Confirm diagnosis by CBC, platelet count, platelet function tests, and bone marrow examination. Tests should be ordered to exclude other causes of thrombocytopenia (e.g., lupus erythematosus).
2. First treat with corticosteroids such as prednisone 60 mg/day for 4–6 weeks and gradually taper.
3. If thrombocytopenia recurs after withdrawing corticosteroids, splenectomy should be considered. Consult a hematologist. Splenectomy should also be considered in patients who fail to respond to corticosteroids.
4. Immunosuppressive therapy may be tried if the above measures fail.

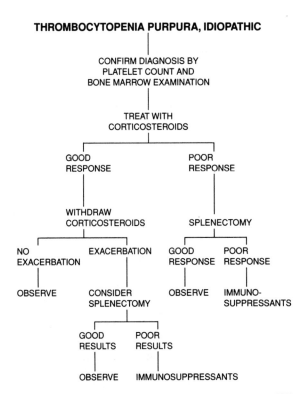

THROMBOCYTOPENIA PURPURA, IDIOPATHIC

THROMBOPHLEBITIS

1. Confirm diagnosis by duplex venous ultrasonography, plethysmography, ^{125}I fibrinogen scan, and venography.
2. *Superficial vein:* Treat with warm saline soaks and elevation. If there is proximal extension, consider anticoagulants.
3. *Deep vein:* Add anticoagulants to above program. Heparin 5000–10,000 units is given initially IV, followed by a continuous infusion of 1000–1500 units/hour. Keep partial thromboplastin time at 1½–2 times the control. When patient recovers, warfarin sodium can be substituted for the heparin.
4. If there is no repeat pulmonary embolism, the patient can be followed with oral anticoagulants for 6 months.
5. If there are repeat pulmonary emboli, consider placing a filter in the inferior vena cava.

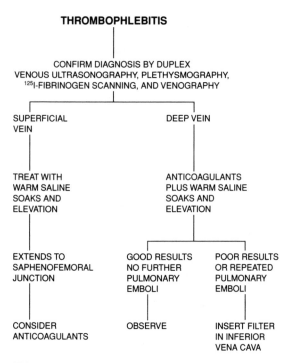

THROMBOPHLEBITIS

CONFIRM DIAGNOSIS BY DUPLEX VENOUS ULTRASONOGRAPHY, PLETHYSMOGRAPHY, ^{125}I-FIBRINOGEN SCANNING, AND VENOGRAPHY

SUPERFICIAL VEIN

DEEP VEIN

TREAT WITH WARM SALINE SOAKS AND ELEVATION

ANTICOAGULANTS PLUS WARM SALINE SOAKS AND ELEVATION

EXTENDS TO SAPHENOFEMORAL JUNCTION

GOOD RESULTS NO FURTHER PULMONARY EMBOLI

POOR RESULTS OR REPEATED PULMONARY EMBOLI

CONSIDER ANTICOAGULANTS

OBSERVE

INSERT FILTER IN INFERIOR VENA CAVA

THROMBOTIC THROMBOCYTOPENIA PURPURA

1. Confirm diagnosis by CBC, platelet count, peripheral blood smears, Coombs' test, and gingival and bone marrow biopsies.
2. Consult a hematologist for evaluation for exchange transfusions or intensive plasmapheresis combined with infusion of fresh plasma.

THYMOMA

1. Confirm diagnosis by chest x-ray and CT scan of the superior mediastinum.
2. Consult a thoracic surgeon for transcervical or transsternal thymectomy.
3. Radiotherapy may be useful in malignant thymoma. Consult a radiotherapist.

THYROIDITIS, SUBACUTE

1. Confirm diagnosis by CBC, sedimentation rate, TSH, and thyroid profile. An RAI uptake and scan may be helpful.
2. Treat inflammation with prednisone 40−60 mg/day for 2 weeks and gradually taper.
3. Treat the thyrotoxicosis with 20−40 mg of propranolol q.i.d.
4. Watch the patient for the development of hypothyroidism and treat accordingly (page 232).

TOURETTE'S SYNDROME

1. Confirm diagnosis by the clinical picture and consultation with a neurologist and/or a psychiatrist.
2. Treatment may be unnecessary in mild cases.
3. In more severe cases, treat with haloperidol beginning at a low dose of 0.25 mg/day and gradually increasing. maximum dose is 8 mg/day. If the drug is to be discontinued, it should be done gradually.
4. Other drugs that may be tried include clonidine, clonazepam, fluphenazine, and pimozide.

TOXOPLASMOSIS

1. Confirm diagnosis by serologic tests or inoculation of blood and body fluids from the patient into the peritoneal cavity of mice.
2. No specific therapy is necessary in the majority of patients unless symptoms persist.
3. Patients with ocular toxoplasmosis and the immunosuppressed patient should be treated with pyrimethamine (200 mg stat, followed by 50–75 mg/day) and sulfadiazine 4–6 g/day in divided doses. Continue therapy for 4–6 weeks. Calcium folinate 10–15 mg/day is also required for 6 weeks. Alternatively, include clindamycin and dapsone.
4. Prevent the disease by eating only adequately cooked meat and avoiding the cat's litter box.

TRACHOMA

1. Confirm diagnosis by Giemsa staining of conjunctival smears, cell cultures, and *Chlamydia* PCR. A therapeutic trial may establish the diagnosis.
2. Treat with 1–3% tetracycline ophthalmic ointment or drops b.i.d. for 3 months. Alternatively, oral tetracycline 15 mg/kg daily for 2 weeks is effective.
3. An ophthalmologist should be consulted for surgical treatment of corneal opacities and scarring of the eyelids.

TRANSFUSION REACTION

1. Confirm diagnosis by repeat type and cross match, direct and indirect Coombs' test, CBC, platelet count, PT, PTT, serum haptoglobin, fibrinogen, and quantitative fibrin split products. Consult a hematologist.
2. Stop transfusion.
3. Treat allergic reactions with diphenhydramine 50 mg q.6h. IV or p.o.
4. Treat nonhemolytic febrile reactions with acetaminophen or aspirin. Consult a hematologist.
5. Treat hemolytic transfusion reactions by maintaining diuresis with 5% dextrose and water solutions. If diuresis is inadequate, administer furosemide or 55 g of 20% mannitol infused over 5–10 minutes.
6. If DIC develops, consult a hematologist and start intravenous heparin and consider the use of cryoprecipitate.

TRANSIENT ISCHEMIC ATTACKS

1. Confirm diagnosis by carotid scans, echocardiography, and four-vessel cerebral angiography. MRI angiography may be useful and obviate the need for four-vessel contrast angiography.
2. If there is a surgically correctable lesion, consult a neurosurgeon or a vascular surgeon.
3. If there is no surgically correctable lesion and the patient is not hypertensive, start anticoagulation with heparin and subsequently transfer over to oral anticoagulants (warfarin sodium).
4. If there is significant hypertension, treat with antihypertensive medication and follow with antiplatelet therapy (aspirin).

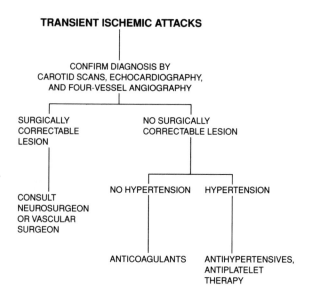

TRICHINOSIS

1. Confirm diagnosis with eosinophil count, muscle enzyme tests, and bentonite flocculation test. Muscle biopsy may be helpful as may other serologic tests. Consult a clinical pathologist.
2. Treat intestinal stage with thiabendazole 22 mg/kg b.i.d. p.o. for 5 days.
3. Treat advanced stage with mebendazole 300 mg t.i.d. p.o. for 3 days and then 500 mg b.i.d. for 10 days. A course of prednisone 40–60 mg/day is given concurrently for 5 days and gradually tapered.

TRIGEMINAL NEURALGIA

1. Confirm diagnosis by clinical picture. Consult a neurologist in confusing cases.
2. First treat with carbamazepine in doses of 100 mg b.i.d. orally and gradually increasing until a response is achieved. The maximum dose is 400 mg t.i.d.
3. If the above drug fails to achieve results, try phenytoin 300–600 mg/day.
4. If the above drugs are ineffective, add baclofen 10–20 mg q.i.d.
5. If drug treatment is unsuccessful, refer to a neurosurgeon for microvascular decompression.

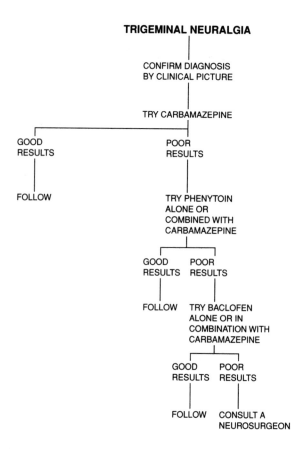

TRIGEMINAL NEURALGIA

CONFIRM DIAGNOSIS
BY CLINICAL PICTURE

TRY CARBAMAZEPINE

GOOD RESULTS

POOR RESULTS

FOLLOW

TRY PHENYTOIN ALONE OR COMBINED WITH CARBAMAZEPINE

GOOD RESULTS | POOR RESULTS

FOLLOW | TRY BACLOFEN ALONE OR IN COMBINATION WITH CARBAMAZEPINE

GOOD RESULTS | POOR RESULTS

FOLLOW | CONSULT A NEUROSURGEON

TRYPANOSOMIASIS

1. Confirm diagnosis by examination of Giemsa-stained thick and thin blood smears and mouse inoculation of blood or tissue fluid or culture of blood on special media. In African trypanosomiasis, fluid expressed from the chancre may be examined under light microscopy for the motile organisms.

2. *African trypanosomiasis:* Treat with suramin, pentamidine, organic arsenicals, and eflornithine, depending on the stage of the disease and whether it is East African or West African type. Consult the CDC or a parasitologist for guidance.

3. *Chagas' disease:* Treat with nifurtimox 8−10 mg/kg daily in four divided doses. Continue treatment for 90−120 days. Contact the CDC to obtain the drug and get guidance in dosage.

TUBERCULOSIS

1. Confirm diagnosis by x-rays and smears and cultures of sputum, urine, body fluids, or tissues of patients suspected of the disease. Tuberculin tests, serological tests, and guinea pig inoculation may be utilized.
2. There are many treatment programs for tuberculosis. The following three are suggested by the author.
   a. Isoniazid 300 mg and rifampin 600 mg daily for 9–12 months.
   b. Isoniazid 300 mg and ethambutol 15 mg/kg daily for 12–18 months.
   c. Isoniazid 300 mg and thioacetazone 150 mg daily for 12–18 months.

   Consult an infectious disease specialist for guidance in therapy.
3. *Prevention:* Treat patients with positive tuberculin tests who may have been infected with tuberculosis with isoniazid 300 mg daily for up to 1 year.

TUBEROUS SCLEROSIS

1. Confirm diagnosis by family history, clinical picture, skin biopsy, and MRIs.
2. Treat epilepsy as a seizure disorder (page 140).
3. Other treatment is symptomatic. Observe brain tumors for obstruction of the ventricles and treat with neurosurgical intervention.

TULAREMIA

1. Confirm diagnosis by rising titers of agglutinating antibodies.
2. Treat with streptomycin 7.5–10 mg/kg q.12h. for 7–10 days.
3. Alternatively, the disease may be treated with gentamicin 1.7 mg/kg IV or IM q.8h. Tetracycline or chloramphenicol have also been used.
4. *Prevention:* Vaccination may be given to high-risk populations. Contact the CDC for details.

TURNER'S SYNDROME

1. Confirm diagnosis by serum FSH and LH, buccal smear, and chromosomal analysis.
2. Consult a gynecologist for treatment with estrogen at the appropriate chronological age.
3. Consider referral to pediatric endocrinologist for growth hormone therapy.

TYPHOID FEVER

1. Confirm diagnosis with stool, urine, or blood cultures and the Widal test.
2. Treat with chloramphenicol 500 mg IV or p.o. q.4h. Treatment is continued for 14−21 days, but dosage may be reduced if the patient improves.
3. Alternatively, ampicillin in doses of 1−2 grams q.6h. IV may be given or trimethoprim-sulfamethoxazole (160 mg/800 mg) IV or p.o. b.i.d. for 14−28 days.
4. *Chronic carriers:* These are also treated, but the period of treatment is 6 weeks.

TYPHUS, EPIDEMIC

1. Confirm diagnosis by the Weil–Felix reaction and complement-fixation tests.
2. Treat with doxycycline 100 mg b.i.d. for 3–7 days or chloramphenicol 500–1000 mg q.i.d. for 3–7 days.
3. *Prevention:* A vaccine is available. Use DDT to eliminate lice.

ULCERATIVE COLITIS

1. Confirm diagnosis by colonoscopy and biopsy. Barium enema may be helpful. Consult a gastroenterologist.
2. *Mild to moderate cases:*
   a. Treat with sulfasalazine 500 mg b.i.d. and gradually increase until disease is controlled or 4–6 g/day is given.
   b. If the above is ineffective, oral prednisone 45–60 mg/day may be given.
   c. If neither of the above drugs is effective, an immunosuppressant agent may be added.
   d. When all forms of medical therapy are unsuccessful, a colectomy should be considered. Consult a surgeon.
3. Severely ill patients should be begun on corticosteroids immediately, orally or IV (use methylprednisolone 60–100 mg q.6–8h.), and given intravenous alimentation. They can gradually be transitioned to oral steroids and sulfasalazine once the disease is under control.
4. *Toxic megacolon:* These patients are treated with intravenous alimentation, balanced electrolytes and intravenous corticosteroids in large doses for 24–48 hours. If significant improvement does not occur, emergency colectomy should be done.

ULCERATIVE COLITIS

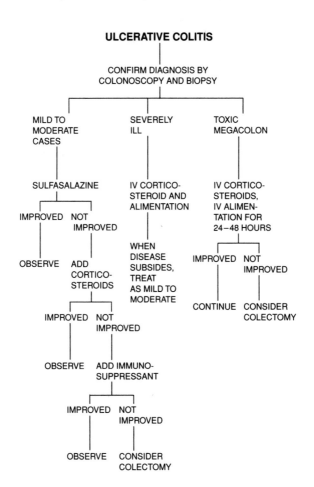

CONFIRM DIAGNOSIS BY
COLONOSCOPY AND BIOPSY

MILD TO MODERATE CASES

SULFASALAZINE

IMPROVED → OBSERVE

NOT IMPROVED → ADD CORTICO-STEROIDS

IMPROVED → OBSERVE

NOT IMPROVED → ADD IMMUNO-SUPPRESSANT

IMPROVED → OBSERVE

NOT IMPROVED → CONSIDER COLECTOMY

SEVERELY ILL

IV CORTICO-STEROID AND ALIMENTATION

WHEN DISEASE SUBSIDES, TREAT AS MILD TO MODERATE

TOXIC MEGACOLON

IV CORTICO-STEROIDS, IV ALIMEN-TATION FOR 24–48 HOURS

IMPROVED → CONTINUE

NOT IMPROVED → CONSIDER COLECTOMY

URINARY TRACT INFECTION

1. Confirm diagnosis with urinalysis, urine culture, and colony count.
2. Rule out obstructive uropathy and systemic disease.
3. In males do urethral smear and prostatic massage.
4. *Urethral smear with or without prostate massage is positive:*
   a. Trimethoprim-sulfamethoxazole double strength twice daily for 6–12 weeks.
   b. Demeclocycline 100 mg b.i.d. for 6 weeks.
5. *Urethral smear with prostatic massage is negative:* Study further with IVP, voiding cystogram, ultrasound or consult urologist.
6. *In females with cystitis only:* Single dose of amoxicillin 3 g orally or single dose of two double-strength trimethoprim sulfamethoxazole tablets.
7. *In females with pyelonephritis:* Hospitalize for IV antibiotics.
   a. Amoxicillin 1 g q.8h. or ampicillin 1 g q.6h. IV for 10–14 days.
   b. Trimethoprim-sulfamethoxazole double-strength tablets twice a day for 14 days.
   c. Rule out obstructive uropathy. Consult a urologist if infection persists.
8. *In children:*
   a. Rule out obstructive uropathy with sonography, voiding cystogram, and IVP; consult a urologist.
   b. If febrile, hospitalize.
   c. Gentamicin 3–5 mg/kg daily IV.
   d. Ampicillin 1 g IV q.6h.
   e. Continue treatment 14 days. May switch to oral therapy once afebrile for 24 hours.

URINARY TRACT INFECTION

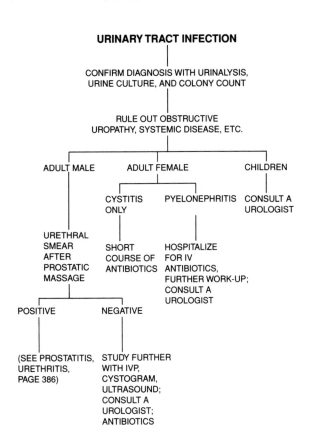

CONFIRM DIAGNOSIS WITH URINALYSIS,
URINE CULTURE, AND COLONY COUNT

RULE OUT OBSTRUCTIVE
UROPATHY, SYSTEMIC DISEASE, ETC.

ADULT MALE   ADULT FEMALE   CHILDREN

                CYSTITIS   PYELONEPHRITIS   CONSULT A
                ONLY   UROLOGIST

URETHRAL
SMEAR   SHORT   HOSPITALIZE
AFTER   COURSE OF   FOR IV
PROSTATIC   ANTIBIOTICS   ANTIBIOTICS,
MASSAGE   FURTHER WORK-UP;
                             CONSULT A
                             UROLOGIST

POSITIVE   NEGATIVE

(SEE PROSTATITIS, STUDY FURTHER
URETHRITIS,   WITH IVP,
PAGE 386)   CYSTOGRAM,
                   ULTRASOUND;
                   CONSULT A
                   UROLOGIST;
                   ANTIBIOTICS

URTICARIA

1. Confirm diagnosis by family history, clinical picture, serum IgE, and skin testing.
2. Treat with H1 class antihistamines such as cyproheptadine and hydroxyzine. Combinations of H1 and H2 antihistamines and sympathomimetic agents are even better.
3. Inborn C11 NH deficiency can be corrected by attenuated androgens. Consult an allergist for assistance.

UTERINE FIBROIDS

1. Confirm diagnosis by ultrasonography, CT scans of the pelvis, and laparoscopy.
2. Asymptomatic uterine fibroids may be treated by observation unless they are pedunculated and subject to acute strangulation.
3. Hysterectomy is the treatment of choice for large or symptomatic fibroids. Consult a gynecologist.

VAGINITIS

1. Confirm diagnosis by vaginal smear and culture and microscopic examination of a saline and KOH preparation. Cultures are available for *Trichomonas vaginalis* and also *Candida.* Evaluate for diabetes.
2. *Bacterial vaginitis:* Treat with metronidazole 500 mg b.i.d. for 7 days. Alternatively, clindamycin 300 mg b.i.d. may be administered for 7 days.
3. *Candidiasis:* Treat with intravaginal miconazole or clotrimazole creams nightly for 7 days. Treatment may need to be given for 14 days in double doses. A single dose of fluconazole 150 mg given orally may be just as effective and more convenient.
4. *Trichomoniasis:* Treat with single oral dose of 2 g of metronidazole. This may be repeated. Alternatively, a 7-day course of 500 mg b.i.d. may be given.
5. *Gonorrhea:* See page 504.

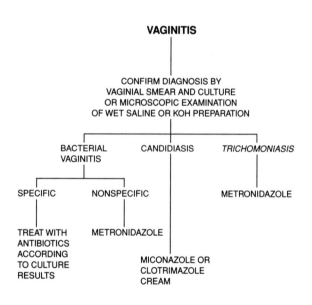

VARICELLA

1. Confirm diagnosis by Tzanck smear or serologic tests.
2. For most cases, treatment is symptomatic because the disease is self-limited.
3. In the immunocompromised, most physicians administer specific zoster immune globulin, varicella-zoster immune globulin, or zoster immune plasma. Consult an infectious disease specialist.
4. Adolescents and adults may need to be given acyclovir 800 mg p.o. five times a day for 5–7 days.

VARICOSE VEINS

1. Confirm diagnosis by clinical picture and venography.
2. Treat medically with support hose, Jobst stockings, and work modification.
3. Smaller varicosities may be treated with sclerosing solutions (sodium morrhuate, etc.) Larger varicosities can be treated with ligation and stripping. Consult a surgeon.

VARIOLA

1. Confirm diagnosis by viral isolation from skin lesions, oropharynx, conjunctiva, and urine. Serological tests are also useful. Global eradication of the disease has been accomplished.
2. Since this is a viral disease, no specific therapy is available. However, vaccination and vaccinia immune globulin administered early in the disease can modify its course.

VENEREAL DISEASE

1. Confirm diagnosis by smear culture, dark-field examination, skin tests, biopsy, and immunologic tests.
2. *Chancroid:* Erythromycin 500 mg q.i.d. p.o. for 1 week. Alternatives are ceftraxone 250 mg IM as a single dose and Bactrim DS 1 tablet b.i.d. p.o. for 5–7 days.
3. *Gonorrhea:* Ceftriaxone 125 mg IM, followed by doxycycline 100 mg b.i.d. p.o. for 7 days. Alternatives are:
   a. Spectinomycin 2 g IM as single dose.
   b. Ciprofloxacin 500 mg p.o. as a single dose.
4. *Gonorrhea disseminated:* Cefotaxime 1 g IM or IV daily until 48 hours after symptoms resolve. Then cefixime 400 mg p.o. for 7–10 days. Alternatives are cefotaxime and ceftizoxime.
5. *Chalmydia trachomatis:* Uncomplicated: Doxycycline 100 mg b.i.d. p.o. for 7 days. Complicated: Continue same antibiotic for 14 days. Alternatives: Azithromycin 1 g as a single dose; tetracycline 500 mg q.i.d. for 7 days.
6. For more discussion see specific disease titles.

VIRAL MYELITIS

1. Confirm diagnosis by spinal fluid analysis, viral isolation, and acute and chronic phase sera for viral serology.
2. Therapy is supportive because there is no specific therapy available.

VISCERAL AND OCULAR LARVA MIGRANS

1. Confirm diagnosis by ELISA for toxocaral antibodies.
2. Presently the available antihelminthic drugs do not seem to alter the disease.

VON WILLEBRAND'S DISEASE

1. Confirm diagnosis by prolonged bleeding time, reduced plasma vWF concentration, reduced ristocetin cofactor activity, and low Factor VIII activity.
2. Treat with cryoprecipitate or the vasopressin analogue 1-desamino-8-D-arginine vasopressin. Consult a hematologist for guidance.

WARTS

1. Confirm diagnosis by clinical evaluation. When in doubt, consult a dermatologist.
2. Treat lesions of the head, neck, trunk, and proximal extremities with electrodesiccation.
3. Repeated applications of liquid nitrogen or liquid CO_2 is effective for thick warts of the hands and feet. Consult a dermatologist.
4. Genital and anal warts may be treated with podophyllin 20% solution in tincture of benzoin. Apply once weekly until warts are gone. This should be done as an in office procedure.

WEGENER'S GRANULOMATOSIS

1. Confirm diagnosis by lung biopsy, upper airway biopsy, and renal biopsy. Elevated titers of anti-neutrophil cytoplasmic antibodies (ANCAs) support the diagnosis.
2. Initially treat with prednisone 1 mg/kg daily and cyclophosphamide 2 mg/kg daily. After the first month, prednisone is tapered and continued on alternate days for 6 months. Continue cyclophosphamide indefinitely until a remission is well established. Consult an oncologist for guidance.
3. Alternatively, azathioprine can be tried.

WERNICKE'S ENCEPHALOPATHY

1. Confirm diagnosis by clinical evaluation and response to therapy. History of alcoholism is helpful.
2. Treat with intravenous thiamine 50 mg. Follow up with oral doses of thiamine and multiple vitamins daily.

WHIPPLE'S DISEASE

1. Confirm diagnosis by small bowel biopsy.
2. Treat with trimethoprim-sulfamethoxazole (160 mg/800 mg) b.i.d. for 1 year. Follow the disease with repeat small bowel biopsies.

YAWS

1. Confirm diagnosis by dark-field examination, RPR, and FTA-ABS test.
2. Treat with 2.4 million units of benzathine penicillin G in adults, and use half that dose in children.
3. In patients who are allergic to penicillin, tetracycline may be used.

YELLOW FEVER

1. Confirm diagnosis by viral isolation from blood and serologic tests.
2. Treatment is symptomatic.
3. *Prevention:* A vaccine is available.

ZOLLINGER–ELLISON SYNDROME

1. Confirm diagnosis by increased serum gastrin levels. For borderline cases, provocative tests such as the secretin injection test and calcium infusion test are available. Consult a gastroenterologistm or endocrinologist.
2. Treat with omeprazole and H2 antagonists.
3. Location and complete resection of the gastrinoma is the most desirable therapy. Consult a specialist in this disease.

INDEX

A

Abdomen, acute, cause of, 6–7
Abscess
  cerebral, 68
  epidural, 139
  liver, 261
  perinephric, 346
  subdiaphragmatic, 461
Acne, 2–3
Acoustic neuroma, 4
Acquired immunodeficiency syndrome, *see* AIDS
Actinomycosis, 5
Acute abdomen, cause of, 6–7
Adenoma
  bronchial, 39
  pituitary, 364–65
Adrenal insufficiency, 8
Adrenogenital syndrome, 9
Agammaglobulinemia, congenital, 10
Agnogenic myeloid metaplasia, 11
AIDS, 12
  prophylaxis, 12
Alcaptonuria, 13
Alcoholic cirrhosis, 84
Alcoholism, 14
Aldosteronism, primary, 15
Allergic rhinitis, 16
Alpha-1 antitrypsin deficiency, 17
Alveolar proteinosis, pulmonary, 393
Alzheimer's disease, 18
Amebiasis, 19
Amphotericin B, administration of, 33
Ampulla of Vater, carcinoma of, 50
Amyloidosis, 20
Anemia
  aplastic, 24
  hemolytic, acquired, 194
  nutritional, 316–17
  pernicious, 351
  sickle cell, 444
Aneurysm
  aortic, 22–23
  cerebral, 69–70
  angina pectoris, *see* coronary insufficiency

Anthrax, 21
  prophylaxis, 21
Antitrypsin, alpha-1, deficiency, 17
Aortic aneurysm, 22–23
  prognosis, 22
Aplastic anemia, 24
Apnea, sleep, 448–49
Appetite suppressants, for obesity, 318
Arrhythmias, cardiac, 61–62
Arteritis, temporal, 469
Arthritis
  osteoarthritis, 322–323
  rheumatoid, 417–18
  septic, 439
Ascaris lumbricoides, 25
Asthma, 26–27
Ataxias, hereditary, 202

B
Bacterial endocarditis, subacute, 460
Balantidiasis, 28
Basilar artery insufficiency, 29
Bell's palsy, 30
Benign intracranial hypertension, 390
Beriberi, 31
Biliary cirrhosis, 32
Blastomycosis, 33
Boeck's sarcoid, 429
Bornholm's disease, 34
Botulism, 35
Bowel, irritable bowel syndrome, 242
Brachial plexus neuropathy, 36
Brain tumors, selected, 37–38
Breast, carcinoma of, 51–52
Bronchial adenoma, 39
Bronchial asthma, 26–27
Bronchiectasis, 40
Bronchitis, acute, 41
Brucellosis, 42
Bursitis, 43

C
Carbon monoxide poisoning, 46
Carbon tetrachloride poisoning, 47
Carbuncles, 48
Carcinoid syndrome, 49
Carcinoma
  of ampulla of Vater, 50
  of breast, 51–52

of cervix, 53
of colon, 54
of endometrium, 55
of esophagus, 147
of lung, 56
of ovary, 57, 333
of pancreas, 58
of prostate, 382–83
of skin, 447
of stomach, 44–45
Cardiac arrest, 59–60
Cardiac arrhythmias, 61–62
Cardiomyopathy, 63–64
Carpal tunnel syndrome, 65
Cat-scratch disease, 66
Celiac disease, *see* malabsorption syndrome, 271
Cellulitis, 67
Cerebral abscess, 68
Cerebral aneurysm, 69–70
Cerebral embolism, 71–72
Cerebral infarction, 73
Cerebral thrombosis, 73
Cervical disk, herniated, 205–06
Cervical spondylosis, 74–75
Cervicitis, 76
Cervix, carcinoma of, 53
Chancroid, 77
Cholangiocarcinoma, 78
Cholangitis, 79
Cholecystitis, 80
Choledocholithiasis, 81
Cholelithiasis, 80
Cholera, 82
Choriocarcinoma, 83
Chronic obstructive Lung disease, *see* Emphysema
Cirrhosis
   alcoholic, 84
   biliary, 32
Cluster headaches, 214
Coccidiomycosis, 85–86
   granulomatous, 406
Colitis, ulcerative, 494–95
Collagen disease, 108, 264, 344
Colon, carcinoma of, 54
Coma, diabetic, 113–14
Congenital heart disease, 89–90
Congestive heart failure, 187–88
Conjunctivitis, 87–88
Constipation, 91
Coronary insufficiency, 92–94
   drugs, dosage, 92

Creutzfeldt-Jakob disease, 95
Cryptococcosis, 96
Cushing's syndrome, 96–97
Cutaneous larva migrans, 99
Cysticercosis, 101
Cystic fibrosis, 100
Cystinosis, 102
Cystinuria, 103
Cytomegalovirus infection, 104

D
Dementia, 18
Dengue fever, 105
Depression, 106–07
  dosages of antidepressant drugs, 106
Dermatitis, allergic, stasis, 457, *see* eczema
Dermatomyositis, 108
Diabetes insipidus, 109
Diabetes mellitus, 110–12
  dosages of oral hypoglycemic agents,
    110
  insulin, giving, 111
Diabetic coma, 113–14
Digitalis intoxication, 115
Diphtheria, 116
  dosage of drugs, 116
  prevention, 116
Diphyllobothrium latum, 117
Disk, herniated
  cervical, 205–06
  lumbar, 207–08
Diverticular disease, 118–19
Down's syndrome, 120
Dracunculiasis, 121
Dressler's syndrome, 122
Drug intoxication, 123
Drug reactions, 124
Dubin-Johnson syndrome, 125

E
Eaton-Lambert syndrome, 126
Echinococcosis, 127
Eclampsia, 380
Ectopic pregnancy, 128
Eczema, 129–30
Ehlers-Danlos syndrome, 131
Elliptocytosis, hereditary, 203
Embolism
  cerebral, 71–72

mesenteric artery, 289
pulmonary, 394–95
Emphysema, 132–33
Empyema of lung, 134
Encephalitis, viral, 135
Encephalomyelitis, acute disseminated, 136
Encephalopathy, Wernicke's, 510
Endocarditis, bacterial, subacute, 460
Endometrium, carcinoma of, 55
Enteritis, regional, 406
Eosinophilic pneumonia, 137
Epididymitis, 138
Epidural abscess, 139
Epilepsy
  idiopathic, 140–42
    dosages of AED's, 140–41
  status, 143
Erysipelas, 144
Erythema
  multiforme, 145
  nodosum, 146
Esophagitis, reflux, 404
Esophagus
  carcinoma, 147
  varices, 148–49
Essential hypertension, 150–51
Extradural hematoma, 152

F
Fabry's disease, 153
Familial Mediterranean fever, 154
Familial periodic paralysis, 155
Fanconi syndrome, 156
Fibroids, uterine, 499
Fibromyalgia, 157
Fibrosis, pulmonary, idiopathic, 235
Filariasis, 158
Fracture, 159
Fungal infections, of skin, 160–61
  anti-fungal preparations, 160
Furuncles, 48

G
Galactosemia, 162
Gas gangrene, 163
Gastritis, 164
Gastroenteritis, 165–66
Gaucher's disease, 167
Giardiasis, 168

Gilbert's disease, 169
Gingivitis, 170
Glanders, 171
Glanzmann's disease, 172
Glaucoma, 173
Glomerulonephritis, 174
Glycogen storage disease, 175
Goiter, diffuse, 176–77
Gonorrhea, 178–79
Goodpasture's disease, 180
Gout, 181
Granuloma inguinale, 182
Granulomatosis
  Langerhans' cell, 247
  Wegener's, 509
Grave's disease, 225–27
Guillain-Barré syndrome, 183

H
Hartnup disease, 184
Head injury, 185–86
Heart failure, 187–88
Heart-related disorders, 61–62, 92–94, 187–189,
    416
Hemangioblastoma, 190
Hematoma
  extradural, 152
  subdural, 462
Hemifacial spasm, 191
Hemochromatosis, 192
Hemoglobin C disease, 193
Hemolytic anemia, acquired, 194
Hemophilia, 195
Hemorrhage, intracranial, 241
Hemorrhagic fever, 196
Hemorrhoids, 197
Hepatitis
  toxic, 198
  viral, 199
Hepatolenticular degeneration, 200
Hepatoma, 201
Hereditary ataxias, 202
Hereditary elliptocytosis, 203
Hereditary spherocytosis, 204
Herniated disk
  cervical, 205–06
    drugs, dosages, 205
  lumbar, 207–08
Herpangina, 209
Herpes simplex, 210

Herpes zoster, 211
Hidradenitis suppurativa, 212
Hirschsprung's disease, 213
Histamine cephalalgia, 214
Histiocytosis X, 215
Histoplasmosis, 216
Hodgkin's disease, *see* Lymphoma
Hookworm disease, 217
Huntington's chorea, 218
Hurler's syndrome, 219
Hydrocephalus, 220
Hypernephroma, 221
Hyperparathyroidism, 222
Hypersensitivity pneumonitis, 223
Hypersensitivity vasculitis, 224
Hypertension, essential, 150–51
Hyperthyroidism, 225–27
Hypertrophy, prostatic, 384–85
Hypoparathyroidism, 228–29
Hypopituitarism, 230–31
Hypotension, postural, idiopathic, 234
Hypothyroidism, 232–33

I

Idiopathic postural hypotension, 234
Idiopathic pulmonary fibrosis, 235
Impetigo, 236
Impingement syndrome, 237
Infarction, cerebral, 73
Infectious mononucleosis, 238
Influenza, 239
Insulinoma, 240
Intestinal tumors, small, 450
Intracranial hemorrhage, 241
Irritable bowel syndrome, 242
Islet cell tumor, *see* Insulinoma

K

Kala-Azar, 243
Kidney, polycystic disease, 375
Klinefelter's syndrome, 244
Korsakoff's syndrome, 245

L

Lactase deficiency, 246
Langerhans' cell granulomatosis, 247
Larva migrans
  cutaneous, 99
  visceral, ocular, 506

Laryngitis, acute, 248
Lead intoxication, 249
Legionnaire's disease, 250
Leishmaniasis, cutaneous, 251
Leprosy, 252
Leptospirosis, 253
Leriche syndrome, 254
Leukemia, 255–56
Lichen planus, 257
Lipoproteinemias, 258–59
  dosages of drugs used to lower cholesterol, 258
Listeriosis, 260
Liver abscess, 261
Liver failure, 262
Lung
  carcinoma of, 56
  disease of, 263
  empyema of, 134
Lupus erythematosus, 264
Lyme disease, 265
Lymphangitis, 266
Lymphogranuloma venereum, 267
Lymphoma, 268
Lysosomal storage disease, 269

M

Macroglobulinemia, 270
Malabsorption syndrome, 271–72
Malaria, 273–74
  prophylaxis, 273
Mallory-Weiss tear, 275
Marfan's syndrome, 276
Mastocytosis, systemic, 466
Mastoiditis, 277
McArdle's syndrome, 278
McCune-Albright syndrome, 279
Meckle's diverticulum, 280
Mediastinitis, 281
Mediterranean fever, familial, 154
Melanoma, 282
Meniere's disease, 283
Meningitis, 284–85
  prophylaxis, 284
Meningococcemia, 286
Menopause, 287–88
Mesenteric artery insufficiency, 289
Methemoglobinemia, 290
Migraine, 291–92
Milroy's disease, 293
Mitral valvular disease, 294–95

Moniliasis, 500
Mucormycosis, 296
Multiple myeloma, 297
Multiple sclerosis, 298
Mumps, 299
Muscular atrophy, peroneal, 352
Muscular dystrophy, 300
Myasthenia gravis, 301–2
Myelitis, viral, 505
Myeloid metaplasia, agnogenic, 11
Myocardial infarction, 303–04
Myotonia atrophica, 305
Myxedema, 232–233

N
Narcolepsy, 306
Nephrolithiasis, 307–08
Nephritis, *see* Glomerulonephritis
Nephrotic syndrome, idiopathic, 309–10
Neuralgia, trigeminal, 486
Neuritis, optic, 319
Neuroblastoma, 311
Neurofibromatosis, 312
Neuroma
  acoustic, 4
  traumatic, 313
Neuropathy
  brachial plexus, 36
  peripheral, 347–49
  peroneal, 353
Niemann-Pick disease, 314
Nocardiosis, 315
Nutritional anemia, 316–17

O
Obesity, 318
  appetite suppressants, 318
Ochronosis, 13
Ocular larva migrans, 506
Oligophrenia, phenylpyruvic, 359
Optic neuritis, 319
Orchitis, 320
Oroya fever, 321
Osteoarthritis, 322–23
  dosages of drugs used to combat osteoarthritis,
    323
Osteogenesis imperfecta, 324
Osteogenic sarcoma, 324
Osteomalacia, 326

Osteomyelitis, 327
Osteopetrosis, 328
Osteoporosis, 329–30
  oral calcium preparations, dosages, 329
Otitis externa, 331
Otitis media, 322
Ovarian cancer, 333
Ovary
  carcinoma of, 57
  polycystic syndrome, 376

P

Paget's disease, 334
Pancreas, carcinoma of, 58
Pancreatitis, 335–36
Panniculitis, acute, 337
Paralysis, periodic, familial, 155
Paralysis agitans, 338–39
Pellagra, 340
Pemphigus vulgaris, 341
Peptic ulcer, 342–43
Periarteritis nodosa, 344
Pericarditis, 345
Perinephric abscess, 346
Periodic paralysis, familial, 155
Peripheral neuropathy, 347–49
  dosages of drugs used in, 347–48
Peritonitis, 350
Pernicious anemia, 351
Peroneal muscular atrophy, 352
Peroneal neuropathy, 353
Pertussis, 354
Peutz-Jeghers syndrome, 355
Peyronie's disease, 356
Pharyngitis, 357
Pharyngoconjunctival fever, 358
Phenylpyruvic oligophrenia, 359
Pheochromocytoma, 360
Phlebotomus fever, 361
Pinealoma, 362
Pinworm disease, 363
Pituitary adenoma, 364–65
Pityriasis rosea, 366
Plague, 367
Pneumoconiosis, 368
Pneumocystis carinii, 369
Pneumonia, 370–71
  eosinophilic, 137
Pneumonitis, hypersensitivity, 223
Pneumothorax, 372–73

Poisoning
  carbon monoxide, 46
  carbon tetrachloride, 47
Poliomyelitis, 374
  prophylaxis, 374
Polychondritis, relapsing, 409
Polycystic kidney disease, 375
Polycystic ovary syndrome, 376
Polycythemia vera, 377
Polymyalgia rheumatica, 378
Porphyria, 379
Postural hypotension, idiopathic, 234
Preeclampsia-eclampsia, 380
Pregnancy, ectopic, 128
Premenstrual tension syndrome, 381
Prophylaxis, 239
Prostatic carcinoma, 382–83
Prostatic hypertrophy, 384–85
Prostatitis, 386
Proteinosis, alveolar, pulmonary, 393
Pseudogout, 387
Pseudohypoparathyroidism, 388
Pseudo-pseudohypoparathyroidism, 389
Pseudotumor cerebri, 390
Psittacosis, 391
Psoriasis, 392
Pulmonary alveolar proteinosis, 393
Pulmonary embolism, 394–95
Pulmonary fibrosis, idiopathic, 235
Pyelonephritis, 396
Pyloric stenosis, congenital, 397
Pyridoxine deficiency, 398

Q
Q-fever, 399

R
Rabies, 400
Rat-bite fever, 401
Raynaud's disease, 402
Reflex sympathetic dystrophy, 403
Reflux esophagitis, 404
Refsum's disease, 405
Regional enteritis, 406
Reiter's syndrome, 407
Relapsing fever, 408
Relapsing polychondritis, 409
Renal calculus, 307–08

Renal failure
  acute, 410–11
  chronic, 412–13
Renal vein thrombosis, 414
Retinal artery occlusion, 415
Rheumatic fever, 416
Rheumatoid arthritis, 417–18
Rheumatoid spondylitis, 419
Rhinitis, allergic, 16
Riboflavin deficiency, 420
Rickets, 421
Rickettsialpox, 422
Rocky Mountain spotted fever, 423
Rubella, 424
Rubeola, 425

S
Salmonellosis, 426–27
Salpingitis, 428
Sarcoidosis, 429
Sarcoma, osteogenic, 324
Scabies, 430
Scalenus anticus syndrome *see* Thoracic outlet
    syndrome
Scarlet fever, 431
Schilder's disease, 432
Schistosomiasis, 433
Schizophrenia, 434
Scleroderma, 435
Sclerosis, tuberous, 489
Scrub typhus, 436
Scurvy, 437
Seborrheic dermatitis, 438
Senile dementia, *see* Alzheimer's disease 439
Septic arthritis, 439
Septicemia, 440
Serum sickness, 441
Shigellosis, 442
Shy-Drager syndrome, 443
Sickle cell anemia, 444
Sinusitis, 445
Sjögren's syndrome, 446
Skin, fungal infections of, 160–61
Skin cancer, 447
Sleep apnea, 448–49
Snake bite, 451
Spastic colitis, *see* Irritable bowel syndrome
Spasmotic torticollis, 452
Spherocytosis, hereditary, 204
Spinal cord tumor, 453

Spondylitis, rheumatoid, 419
Spondylosis, cervical, 74–75
Sporotrichosis, 454
Sprains, common, 455–56
Stasis dermatitis, 457
Stein-Leventhal syndrome, 376
Stenosis, pyloric, congenital, 397
Stomach, cancer of, 44–45
Strongyloidiasis, 458
Sturge-Weber syndrome, 459
Subacute bacterial endocarditis, 460
Subdiaphragmatic abscess, 461
Subdural hematoma, 462
Sulfhemoglobinemia, 290
Syphilis, 463–64
Syringomyelia, 465
Systemic mastocytosis, 466

T
Takayasu's disease, 467
Tapeworm disease, 468
Temporal arteritis, 469
Testicular tumors, 470
Tetanus, 471
Thalassemia, 472
Thoracic outlet syndrome, 473
Thromboangiitis obliterans, 474
Thrombocytopenia purpura
   idiopathic, 475
   thrombotic, 477
Thrombophlebitis, 476
Thrombosis
   basilar artery, 29
   cerebral, and infarction, 73
   mesenteric artery, 289
   renal vein, 414
   terminal aorta, see Leriche syndrome
Thrombotic thrombocytopenia purpura, 477
Thymoma, 478
Thyroiditis, subacute, 479
Tic douloureux, 486
TIA, see Transient ischemic attack
Tonsillitis, 357
Torticollis, spasmotic, 452
Tourette's syndrome, 480
Toxic hepatitis, 198
Toxoplasmosis, 481
Trachoma, 482
Transfusion reaction, 483
Transient ischemic attack (TIA), 484

Traumatic neuroma, 313
Trichinosis, 485
Trigeminal neuralgia, 486
Trypanosomiasis, 487
Tuberculosis, 488
Tuberous sclerosis, 489
Tularemia, 490
Turner's syndrome, 491
Typhoid fever, 492
Typhus, epidemic, 493

U
Ulcer, peptic, 342–43
Ulcerative colitis, 494–95
Urinary tract infection, 496–97
Urticaria, 498
Uterine fibroids, 499

V
Vaginitis, 500
Valley fever, *see* Coccidiomycosis
Varicella, 501
Varices, esophageal, 148–49
Varicose veins, 502
Variola, 503
Vasculitis, hypersensitivity, 224
Venereal disease, 504
Viral encephalitis, 135
Viral hepatitis, 199
Viral myelitis, 505
Visceral larva migrans, 506
Vitamin deficiency, 326, 421, 437
Von Gierke's disease, 175
Von Willebrand's disease, 507

W
Warts, 508
Wegener's granulomatosis, 509
Weil's disease, 253
Wernicke's encephalopathy, 510
Whipple's disease, 511

Y
Yaws, 512
Yellow fever, 513

Z
Zollinger-Ellison syndrome, 514